Peptide Therapy

A Step-by-Step Guide for Unlocking The Secrets to Longevity, Vitality, Enhanced Cognitive Function, Rapid Muscle Recovery, Optimal Health, and Anti-Aging in 60 Days

Terry Riccardi MD

Disclaimer

The information provided in this book, 'Peptide Therapy: A Step-by-Step Guide for Unlocking The Secrets to Longevity, Vitality, Enhanced Cognitive Function, Rapid Muscle Recovery, Optimal Health, and Anti-Aging in 60 Days', is for educational and informational purposes only. It is not intended as a substitute for professional medical advice, diagnosis, or treatment. Always consult your healthcare provider before starting any new health regimen, including peptide therapy, to ensure it is safe and appropriate for your individual health needs. The author and publisher assume no responsibility or liability for any potential side effects, complications, or damages resulting from the use or misuse of the information in this book. All efforts have been made to ensure the accuracy of the information, but healthcare practices and peptide therapies may evolve over time. Readers are encouraged to verify any health-related information and work with a qualified professional to address their personal health concerns.

Table of Contents

Introduction...vii

Part 1: Peptide Science Simplified

- The Basics of Peptides...3
- How Peptides Enhance Muscle Recovery and Cognitive Function...9
- The Most Effective Peptides for Health Optimization   17

Part 2: The 60-Day Peptide Therapy Blueprint

- Preparing for Your 60-Day Journey................................. 27
- Weeks 1-2: Starting Strong with Peptide Integration....   37
- Weeks 3-4: Enhancing Muscle Recovery and Cognitive Functions...45
- Weeks 5-6: Longevity and Energy Maximization............. 51
- Weeks 7-8: Finalizing Your 60-Day Transformation....... 59

Part 3: Addressing Skepticism and Myths

- Debunking Myths About Peptide Therapy....................... 73
- Safety Concerns and How to Use Peptides Responsibly 79

Part 4: Lifestyle Strategies to Maximize Peptide Effectiveness

- Nutrition for Longevity and Recovery............................. 89
- The Importance of Sleep and Stress Management....... 99
- Exercise Plans Tailored to Peptide Therapy.................. 107

Part 5: Long-Term Health and Future Applications

- Maintaining Your Results for Life 117
- Innovations in Peptide Therapy.................................... 121

Conclusion

- Your 60-Day Transformation: What's Next? 127

Appendices

- Meal Plan and Exercise Templates 132
- Glossary of Key Terms in Peptide Science 135

Introduction

Why Peptides Are the Future of Health and Longevity

In today's fast-paced world, where everybody is in search of the secret to a longer, healthier, and more youthful life, it just might come from an innovative new frontier: peptide therapy. It involves the use of peptides, which are little chains of amino acids that act as critical messengers inside the body and have become one of the most promising and innovative approaches to enhancing health and well-being.

From improved energy to better cognitive functioning and accelerating the recovery phases of muscles, peptides offer a safe, science-backed, effective method to optimize the natural processes of your body. Unlike so many other treatments that have side effects or risks, peptide therapy works in harmony with your body to help repair, restore, and rejuvenate. With the possible option to revolutionize everything from anti-aging to fitness recovery, peptide therapy protects the future of how we will age gracefully, perform at the top, and live more vibrantly. This book will show you how to tap into that future with crystal-clear, actionable steps one can take today.

The science behind peptides and what they promise

Peptides aren't a fad; they are based on valid scientific studies that keep getting better and better. These small molecules have become important messengers among the body's cells, regulating processes from metabolic rates to tissue repair, hormone production, and much more. Because they are directed at specific receptors within the body, peptides can help speed healing, increase fat burning, enhance immune responses, enhance skin turgor, and also sharpen the mind. Of the exciting areas that peptide therapy encompasses, one is a brand-new way of enhancing longevity and vitality without the harsh side effects often involved with conventional treatments. Whether it be inflammation you hope to reduce, or the need for quality sleep, or the cessation and reversal of the degenerative signs of aging in both your skin and body, peptides offer an effective and natural solution. This book will explain, at a molecular level, how peptides work, but it is also a guide to the most effective peptides available today and how you can take them into your daily routine for maximum impact.

Why This Book Can Change Your Life in 60 Days

Its promise is uncomplicated: in only 60 days, your health, appearance, and overall vitality can dramatically change. When peptide therapy is mixed with certain lifestyle changes, peptide therapy has the potential to create fast-acting and very effective results. The 60-day blueprint of this book targets what's usually the most urgent of your health goals - more energy, quicker muscle recovery, sharper mental acuity, or the secrets to anti-aging.

Unlike so many over-the-top, convoluted wellness plans out there, this one is going to be super simple and evidence-based. Every stage of this program will assist in tapping into the benefits of peptides safely and effectively while folding in small, easily digestible lifestyle modifications that make the therapy even more powerful.

The result? You're going to feel great, and your skin, muscle tone, and overall vitality will visibly improve. This isn't about quick fixes; this is about sustainable health and wellbeing that lasts.

For Whom: The Fitness Enthusiast Looking for Longevity-and the Skeptics Too

This book is a useful tool for a broad-based audience, from the advanced to the beginner, in the realm of fitness and wellness. It will enable fitness enthusiasts who may not have any familiarity with peptide therapy to understand how peptide protocols can help take their recovery and performance to the next level and reduce downtime while building muscle with more ease. Longevity seekers will uncover evidence-based strategies to extend the time of vitality and youthful energy, applying peptides to break visible patterns of aging while boosting cognitive function and physical resilience.

It will help the skeptic by alleviating frequent complaints and myths about peptide therapy, while also presenting powerful evidence and real-life success stories in proving its validity. In this way, you will understand perfectly how peptides work, why they are safe, and just how a game-changer they can be in your pursuit of optimal health. Whether you do it to improve your physical performance, to keep yourself looking and feeling younger, or just to feel better in everyday life, it can provide you with an insight into the necessary tools for lasting change. Read on and discover in this book how peptide therapy does not just involve science, but takes control over life to start living it vigorously, strongly, and youthfully. Welcome to the future of wellness.

Part 1:

Peptide Science Simplified

Chapter 1

The Basics of Peptides

Peptide therapy is proving to be among the most leading-edge methodologies for overall vitality, longevity, and health. To delve deeper into the discussion of specific protocols and benefits, it is important to outline the basics of peptides-how they function in the body, and just why they are so fundamental in cellular regeneration and aging. In this chapter, we will learn what peptides are, their basic function and role in biological processes, and how they can unlock pathways leading to a more vibrant, youthful life.

What are peptides and how do they work in the body?

Peptides are small chains of amino acids, the building blocks of proteins. Whereas proteins contain hundreds of amino acids, peptides comprise between 2 and 50 amino acids. This small size gives peptides unique properties to work as highly specialized messengers that regulate a number of biological activities. Put differently, peptides instruct your body to do certain things, be it repairing muscle tissue, regenerating skin cells, or improving cognitive function.

Fundamentally, peptides interact with cells to turn on pathways leading to various biological effects. These effects range anywhere from increased production of collagen for better skin elasticity to improved recovery post-workout for muscles. The body naturally produces peptides, but some of them are not produced in the same quantity as we get older, adding to the potential for aging.

It is at this point that peptide therapy comes into play: by adding in a peptide that may be absent from or in low supply within the body, natural processes can be stimulated that otherwise would decrease with age.

For example, growth hormone-releasing peptides, like Ipamorelin, stimulate the release of growth hormone needed to develop muscles, burn fat, and repair tissues. Other peptides, like BPC-157, have wound-healing effects and reduce inflammation; thus, these peptides are great during the recovery process of an injury. Since peptides are naturally occurring, their side effects are relatively less compared to other drugs, and they are mostly safe and efficient if used appropriately.

From a boost in the immune system to an improvement in cognitive performance, everything is considered possible with the vast versatility of peptides. The Peptide therapyt can target a very specific physiological function that one feels needs enhancement or repair.

The Role of Peptides in Cellular Regeneration and Repair

As the body grows older, it slowly loses its natural ability to repair and regenerate cells. This manifests as the development of wrinkles, a general feeling of tiredness, or even regression over time with generally inefficient recovery processes after physical overexertion or injury. Peptides are one of the active solutions to this decline, acting directly on the natural cellular repair mechanisms of the body.

Cellular regeneration means the old or damaged cells get replaced by new, healthy ones. Peptides, more so those in the regulation of growth and inflammation, facilitate this very well. Such peptides include BPC-157, which has promised very excellent results in the repair of tissues with the objective of healing muscles, tendons, and ligaments. For that matter, it is one very important peptide for athletes and anybody who wants to recover from injury as soon as possible.

Thymosin Beta-4, or TB-500, is another peptide important in cell migration and growth. It will help support tissue repair and reduce inflammation. Thus, this peptide became very popular in medical studies as it was effective in accelerating wound healing and regenerating damaged tissues in cases of chronic injury.

But peptides don't only help with physical injuries; they help in re-growing vital organs and tissues, which are supposed to aid longevity. For example, mitochondrial peptides like MOTS-c have been shown to improve mitochondrial function, so-called power plants, of our cells. By improving mitochondrial efficiency, peptides like MOTS-c support increased energy generation at the cellular level, improving endurance, physical performance, and the feeling of vitality in general.

Another important function of peptides is the reduction of inflammation, one of the major causes of aging. Chronic inflammation can lead to a plethora of degenerative diseases, such as arthritis, cardiovascular disease, and cognitive decline. In addition to promoting healing, the reduction of inflammation by peptides like

Thymosin Alpha-1 and BPC-157 prevent long-term damage from chronic inflammation.

Why Peptides Are Critical for Longevity and Vitality

When referring to longevity, we are speaking about an extension not only of life but of health span - the amount of time in our lives when we would be healthy both physically and mentally. Longevity is critical because peptides work at the cellular level to rejuvenate your body from the inside out. By facilitating cellular repair, tamping down inflammation, and optimizing a number of key biological processes, peptides offer singular tools for maintaining youthfulness, energy, and overall vitality with increasing age.

One major reason peptides are so essential when it comes to longevity is because of their ability to stimulate growth hormone production. Growth hormone plays an important role in building muscle, regulating body fat metabolism, and tissue repair. Unfortunately, with increasing age, our natural production of growth hormone significantly diminishes, leading to a loss in muscle mass, increased body fat, and, to worsen the situation, recoveries from injuries taking longer periods. This fall in growth hormone production can be opposed by peptides such as CJC-1295 and Ipamorelin, which stimulate the secretion of growth hormone and are believed to give one a younger look, better muscle tone, and recovery rates.

But peptides are not just about physical health. One major concern with someone interested in longevity is cognitive decline, and there are certain peptides that protect and enhance brain function. Neuroprotective peptides include Semax and Selank, which help enhance memory, improve focus, and reduce anxiety. These peptides help improve cognitive function, thus a person can remain sharp mentally with increasing age and spend a better quality life during old age.

Another critical aspect of longevity is reducing the overall burden of stress on the body. Chronic stress accelerates the process of aging and is associated with a range of health problems, including cardiovascular diseases, obesity, and mood disorders. Epitalon is a peptide that has been studied for its anti-aging properties and regulation of the stress response of an individual by balancing melatonin and cortisol production. The harmony of these two hormones helps one to sleep better, have fewer stress episodes, and keep one looking younger.

In conclusion, peptides are revolutionizing the way we approach health and longevity. By enhancing the molecular level of repair and regeneration so naturally performed by the body, peptides could stand as a strong tool in one's quest for gaining long-term vitality, improving physical performance, and further developing cognitive function.

Chapter 2

How Peptides Enhance Muscle Recovery and Cognitive Function

More recently, peptides have gained considerable popularity in medicine, fitness, and wellness because of their huge capabilities with regard to their use for muscle recovery, enhancement of cognitive abilities, and combat against cellular inflammation and stress. This chapter will explore in detail how peptides improve these critical aspects of health and longevity and provide the foundational understanding necessary for the step-by-step process required to unleash their full potential in your daily life.

Muscle Repair: Building Strength and Resilience with Peptides

Muscle recovery plays an important role in the life of any individual who wishes to retain or build better physical health, be it professional athletes, persons who are into regular workouts, or people desiring to age gracefully while remaining active. Muscle damage coupled with its replacement by repair processes is crucial for strength, endurance, and resilience. These damages are minute micro-tears that develop in muscles when they are under stress, as in the case of workouts, and need to heal so that the muscle fibers become stronger. Sometimes recovery is slow, especially as one gets older, and this is where peptides offer game-changing support.

I. Peptide and Muscle Recovery: How the Magic Works

The peptides BPC-157 and TB-500 have gained particular notoriety for their tissue repair and muscle regeneration-enhancing properties. But how exactly do they work?

- **BPC-157** has shown huge promise for healing a wide range of different injuries, ligament, tendon, and muscle damage included; it is a peptide derived from a protein in the stomach. It increases angiogenesis - the formation of new blood vessels, which in turn increases the blood flow to the damaged tissues. The increased blood flow means there is an increase in the supply of nutrients and oxygen to the place of injury, thus increasing the rate of recovery. Moreover, BPC-157 increases the growth factors that expedite cell regeneration, and this enables muscles to heal more and faster.

- **Thymosin Beta-4**, more commonly referred to as TB-500, is another key player in muscle recovery. It works through the regulation of one highly important protein for cell structure and movement called actin, which becomes crucial in such a period as tissue regeneration. TB-500 increases endurance and agility; therefore, it is a great choice for those who wish to prevent injury or recover quicker from tiring activities. The additional anti-inflammatory properties of the peptide increase its overall efficiency by lessening pain and swelling at the affected sites, thus allowing the injury sites to recover more quickly.

These peptides are involved in accelerating muscle healing after an injury and take part in the protection against further damage, which strengthens the tissues and makes them more resilient. In enhancing natural body recovery processes, they are much safer and more natural alternatives than pharmaceutical drugs such as NSAIDs, non-steroidal anti-inflammatory drugs, which can have adverse side effects when used over long periods of time.

II. Applications for Different Groups

- **Athletes and Fitness Enthusiasts:** Most athletes push their bodies beyond the limit, often returning home with frequent injuries and, thus, a constant need for quick recovery. Peptide therapy reduces recovery time, thereby reducing downtime, and one can soon get back to normal working mode. In addition to muscling repair, peptides also prevent scar tissue buildup within the body, thus keeping it more flexible and agile.

- **Older Adults and Age-Related Muscle Loss:** Sarcopenia is an age-related loss of muscle mass and function in older adults, which contributes to the decline in mobility and quality of life. Peptides help to counteract this through their promotion of muscle regeneration, strength improvement, and maintenance of muscle tone with increasing age. For older adults, peptide therapy represents an important means through which individuals can continue to be active, healthy, and independent for a longer period.

Brain Boost: Enhancing Cognitive Functions Through Peptides

Besides the physical benefits, peptides gained a certain popularity for improving one's cognitive function. Sometimes with aging comes the not-so-pleasing cognitive decline, characterized by slower processing, memory loss, and a decrease in focus. Nevertheless, active peptides improve brain health, clear mental fogginess, and can even stop neurodegenerative diseases.

I. **Peptides That Boost Brain Power**

Two peptides that have shown great promise in the ability to enhance cognitive function are Semax and Selank. These neuropeptides work their magic through action on the central nervous system, increasing the activity of the brain in such a manner as to be beneficial for learning, memory retention, and even the regulation of mood.

- **Semax::** This peptide was first synthesized in Russia, initially for the purpose of treating stroke victims, but it has very quickly become renowned for its proficiency in enhancing cognitive function even in healthy individuals. Semax acts to produce BDNF, or brain-derived neurotrophic factor, a protein that takes part in neuroprotective and neurotrophic functions in neuron growth, maintenance, and survival. The improvement of BDNF levels helps to enhance learning capacity and memory retention, along with general brain plasticity- the ability of one's brain to adapt and change according to new information received. Additionally, Semax improves concentration by minimizing fatigue and

decreasing stress levels, which makes it quite useful for high-achievers who often need to think clearly under pressure.

- **Selank:** Another peptide that was developed for its nootropic properties, Selank works by reducing anxiety and improving cognition. The peptide works by modulating neurotransmitter levels, including serotonin and dopamine, both of which are important for mood and clarity. Selank also improves memory and concentration, hence becoming an effective means for keeping one's mental and emotional faculties in order. It is especially helpful for people whose cognitive functions deteriorate under the influence of stress or anxiety because it dispels mental fogginess and sharpens the mind.

II. **Neuroprotection and Long-Term Cognitive Health**

Perhaps what really sets peptides like Semax and Selank apart is their neuroprotective properties. These peptides protect the brain from damages linked to oxidative stress, inflammation, and aging. Oxidative stress is one condition in which there is an imbalance between free radicals and antioxidants within the individual human biological system, thus creating cellular damage. Over time, such kinds of damage may cause neurodegenerative diseases like Alzheimer's and Parkinson's. By reducing inflammation and ultimately leading to the repair of neurons, these peptides can slow down or even completely halt cognitive decline, ensuring better mental health in the future.

Peptide therapy offers better short-term cognitive function and long-term protection against cognitive deterioration. Adding peptides into one's wellness routine is a proactive approach toward enjoying mentally sharp aging.

Cellular Approach for Inflammation and Stress

Of all the factors, chronic inflammation and stress are two of the most important contributors to aging, disease, and loss of vitality. While inflammation is a normal response of an organism (In this case, human) to an injury or illness, when it turns out to be chronic, it can give rise to everything from simple joint pain to serious heart diseases. While long-term stress can amount to catastrophic outcomes on both body and psyche, with the promotion of aging and encouragement of several diseases, peptides hold high power in addressing such problems by reducing inflammation and stress at the cellular level.

I. **Anti-Inflammatory Peptides**

Thymosin Alpha-1 (Tα1) is one such peptide that has enjoyed great application in the treatment of immune diseases and inflammation. Thymosin Alpha-1, therefore, facilitates the action of the T-cells, which are some of the major lymphocytes, identifying and destroying lousy cells. Basically, this peptide bolsters immunity to help one get through infections, but that is not all about this peptide. Additionally, thymosin alpha-1 reduces chronic inflammation by modulating the immune responses. It is, therefore, an excellent choice for patients with autoimmune disorders or those suffering from chronic inflammatory conditions.

Another popularly known peptide is Epitalon, which lowers the level of oxidative stress and normalizes melatonin production. Melatonin is considered a hormone involved in sleep/wake cycles, melatonin has the tendency to reduce inflammation and control the levels of stress. Improving sleep patterns with the help of Epitalon reduces oxidative damage at the cellular level, contributing to general vitality and longevity.

II. **Peptides and Cellular Stress**

Any form of stress, whether it be physical, mental, or emotional, manifests at the cellular level. Chronic stress may eventually lead to malfunction at the cellular level, especially with the progress of aging and the onset of disease. Peptides such as BPC-157 and TB-500 do more than just speed up muscle recovery; they handle the damage to cells brought on by stress. It has also been shown that BPC-157 could reduce damage from oxidative stress, which is one of the major causes of aging and a wide range of chronic diseases. This peptide protects the cells against stress-induced damage, enabling the body to accelerate healing or stay resilient against physical or environmental challenges.

III. **Reducing Inflammation for Longevity and Health**

Peptides attack inflammation and stress at the cellular levels, bringing balance to the body and, slowing aging. Chronic inflammation has been identified as one of the major underlying threats in several diseases such as cardiovascular disease, diabetes, and neurodegenerative diseases. Peptides that reduce inflammation and stress, when incorporated, can make one not only recover quicker but also protect against the long-term damage of chronic inflammation.

Chapter 3

The Most Effective Peptides for Health Optimization

From anti-aging and muscle recovery to cognitive performance, peptide therapy is an incredible tool in the enhancement of health. To get the most from peptides, it's vital to know which peptides are most effective for the various health goals one may have. In this chapter, we will go through the top peptides that promote anti-aging, muscle recovery, and cognitive enhancement and then show how these can be combined in a practical way to give the most effective outcome. Whether you are new to peptides or trying to get your existing peptide regimen optimized, this chapter will help you get the best possible results.

Peptides for Anti-Aging: BPC-157, GHK-Cu, and Thymosin Beta-4

Aging is an inevitable part of life, but peptides definitely will slow down the consequences and sometimes reverse them. Anti-aging science has come a long way, and BPC-157, GHK-Cu, and Thymosin Beta-4 peptides are leading from the front in this revolution-illuminating the body right from its cells.

I. **BPC-157:** Also referred to as the "Body Protection Compound," this is a peptide with great renown for its potent healing and regenerative properties. It enhances the repair of tissues by stimulating the formation of new blood vessels, otherwise known as angiogenesis, and inhibiting inflammation. In relation to anti-aging, BPC-157 plays an important role in tissue healing and increasing cellular repair, even helping in the restoration of internal organs. It also contributes to the digestive system, allowing nutrient absorption and overall vitality. BPC-157 helps the body be in a more youthful state by reducing oxidative stress and promoting anabolic protective processes through the mediation of damaged tissues repair.

II. GHK-Cu: Is a copper-binding peptide that has been studied extensively for its skin rejuvenation properties. GHK-Cu encourages collagen production, a necessary factor in skin elasticity and wrinkling, but it also possesses anti-inflammatory and wound-healing properties. Its DNA-repairing capabilities, oxidative stress reduction, and enhancement of immune function make it one of the most holistic anti-aging peptides available. Beyond skin health, GHK-Cu enhances tissue repair, boosts the immune system, and even modulates gene expression in a manner consistent with longevity.

III. Thymosin Beta-4 (TB-500): This is another peptide generating interest for its regenerative powers. Thymosin Beta-4 plays an important role in tissue repair, immune system modulation, and general cellular health. It works to promote wound healing through cell migration, inhibition of scar tissue formulation, and enhancement of angiogenesis. Thymosin Beta-4 also enhances cellular resistance, and this is of great importance to slowing down the manifestation of visible signs of aging and ensuring optimal functionality of organs. It is highly valued in maintaining muscle tone and reducing the risk of injury with the advancement of the body's age.

Thus, with these peptides incorporated into one's anti-aging regimen, an active effort at slowing down the ticking clock would be realized. They would help preserve youth in the skin through enhanced regeneration of tissues and protection from age-related degeneration.

Rapid Muscle Recovery Peptides: IGF-1, CJC-1295, and Others

Muscle recovery is important for anyone living an active lifestyle-be it a competitive athlete or even someone trying just to stay fit as they age. Peptides like IGF-1, CJC-1295, and other growth hormone secretagogues rank among the most potently used weapons in the toolbox for improving muscle recovery and building strength. Such peptides accelerate the natural healing process of the body, making recoveries from workouts and injuries, even age-related muscle decline, so much quicker.

I. IGF-1 (Insulin-like Growth Factor 1): The most vital peptide in terms of muscle growth and recovery, insulin-like growth factor 1 provides a medium through which the body can increase protein synthesis to grow the size of the muscles. IGF-1 is responsible for enhancing lean body mass, quickening the repair of damaged fibers in muscular tissues following intense workouts, increasing endurance, and hardening the connective tissues, hence reducing the risk of injury. In fact, for athletes and fitness enthusiasts, IGF-1 presents a sure and fast method of gaining muscles, improving performance, and recovering way faster.

II. **CJC-1295: CJC-1295:** Is a growth hormone secretagogue. This means it works to stimulate the production and secretion of growth hormone from the pituitary gland. As one gets older, the level of this naturally occurring growth hormone in the body begins to decrease. CJC-1295 increases muscle repair, strength, and fat loss by boosting growth hormone levels naturally. It also synergistically has a positive interaction with IGF-1 by ensuring muscle growth and recovery, adding much value to the process of fitness optimization.

III. **GHRP- 6(Growth Hormone Releasing Peptide-6):** Growth Hormone Releasing Peptide-6 (GHRP-6): This peptide stimulates growth hormone release. As is expected, like the previous one, this will result in quicker muscle recovery and performance improvement. GHRP 6 suppresses inflammation, which might speed the healing of any injuries and reduce recovery time after strong physical activity. This peptide does much in increasing lean muscle mass, reduction of body fat, and enhancement of the general strength of an individual's body.

IV. **BPC-157:** Although BPC-157 is considered mainly for its repairing properties related to tissues and organs, it does a great deal concerning muscle recovery. It amplifies the repair of torn muscle tissue, reduces inflammation, and quickens the time of recovery after an injury or surgery. In fact, active individuals and athletes alike will benefit from BPC-157 in terms of high performance with less injury-related downtime.

Apart from accelerating the recovery of muscles, these

Ipeptides also contribute to enhancing strength and resilience, making one able to work out harder and recover more quickly. Applied together with an overall health and fitness regimen, it is a safe and effective manner of ensuring peak physical performance on an ongoing basis.

Peptides for Cognitive Enhancement: Cerebrolysin, Dihexa, and More

One of the major worries that comes with aging is cognitive decline. Peptides, however, like Cerebrolysin and Dihexa, raise new hope for the betterment of brain function and protection from neurodegenerative diseases. These peptides have been researched and proven to enhance cognitive performance by enhancing memory and contributing to long-term brain health.

I. **Cerebrolysin:** This neuroprotective peptide enhances memory, learning, and overall cognitive function. Cerebrolysin works its magic by stimulating the growth and repair of neurons, protecting the brain from oxidative stress, and thereby decreasing the chances of neurodegenerative diseases like Alzheimer's. This enables the brain to create new connections, which are quite important in learning and retaining memory. Indeed, Cerebrolysin is something that helps individuals enhance their mental clarity and protect against cognitive decline.

II. **Dihexa:** is a peptide that has been gaining increasing attention due to its action in the improvement of cognitive function. It is known to promote synaptogenesis, which is basically the growth of synapses between neurons.

This is very vital in memory and learning because strong synapses facilitate good communication between brain cells. Cognitive performance was shown to be enhanced with Dihexa administration both in healthy individuals and neurodegenerative patients. This makes it an exceptional tool for anyone desiring the optimization of mental performance by enhancement of brain plasticity.

III. **Selank:** This is a peptide developed to decrease anxiety and enhance cognitive functioning. It works by modulating neurotransmitter activities, such as serotonin and dopamine. It increases memory and learning capabilities while at the same time lowering stress and anxiety; therefore, it can be helpful for those suffering with diminished cognition because of higher levels of stress. Attention and the ability to focus are also improved with the use of Selank, making it useful for those who need to maintain peak mental performance in demanding environments.

Cerebrolysin, Dihexa, and Selank are novel peptides that open the way to enhance cognitive health and prevent brain aging. Whether improving one's memory, sharpening focus, or guarding against neurodegenerative effects, these peptides offer a safe and efficient mode of improving brain functions.

A Practical Guide to Peptide Stacking for Maximum Results

Well, stacking peptides - that is, using more than one peptide simultaneously - is certainly a method by which a little extra efficiency can be wrung out of peptides with peptide therapy, but it's also synergistic. This means targeting different aspects of health to create a peptide protocol that meets your specific goals, whether anti-aging, muscle recovery, or even cognitive enhancement.

I. **Anti-Aging Stacking:** An ideal anti-aging stack can include skin rejuvenation through GHK-Cu, fast tissue repair through BPC-157, and overall regeneration with Thymosin Beta-4. More precisely, it can be useful in keeping the aging process slow, enhancing collagen production, and improving cellular repair so that your body stays young and resilient.

II. **Muscle Recovery Stacking:** Since IGF-1, CJC-1295, and BPC-157 increase muscle recovery, stacking them for professional sports makes one work out better. The risk of injury also decreases. While CJC-1295 increases growth hormone, IGF-1 increases the growth and development of muscles, and BPC-157 increases tissue repair. Thus, such a combination will be ideal for people aiming at ultimate physical performance.

III. **Cognitive Enhancement Stack:** If you are looking out for brain health, the stack of Cerebrolysin, Dihexa, and Selank will facilitate a rise in cognitive performance with enhanced memory and protection from neurodegenerative diseases. Cerebrolysin will support neuron repair, while Dihexa will promote the growth of synapses and Selank will reduce stress and enhance focus. Perfect for those who really want to optimize their mental clarity as well as long-term brain health.

You can target multiple health aspects all at once by strategically stacking peptides together, yielding faster and more complete outcomes. Whether looking to enhance cognitive function, accelerate muscle recovery, or slow the aging process, stacking the right peptides will go a long way toward achieving such goals.

Part 2:

The 60-Day Peptide Therapy Blueprint

Chapter 4

Preparing for Your 60-Day Journey

Beginning a 60-day peptide therapy can be an exciting and transformational process, but you must prepare for it. This chapter aims to walk you through basic steps that will allow you to assess the present state of your health, safely source peptides from reputable sources and set realistic goals regarding health, fitness, and longevity. In so doing, you will ensure that you maximize the benefits of the peptide therapy and guarantee a smooth, efficient process.

Assessing Your Current Health: Key Metrics to Track

One very critical thing, before initiating the peptide therapy, is that a proper evaluation of your present health status should be done. This will be essential for not only creating a baseline from which one can track his or her progress but also for ascertaining that the right peptides selected are required by one's particular health condition. Without it, there would be misguided treatment with the compromising of effectiveness associated with the 60-day journey.

I. Body Composition: Of all the metrics one might watch, body composition-referring to muscle mass versus fat-is rather crucial. Peptide therapy, particularly with peptides such as IGF-1 and CJC-1295, has a reputation for leading to greater lean muscle growth while somewhat lowering fat. Use tools like DEXA scans, bioelectrical impedance scales, or even skinfold calipers to get a proper picture of your body composition.

Your measurements of muscle mass, body fat percentage, and weight will provide a good insight into the effectiveness of the peptides within these 60 days.

- **Why it matters:** Measuring your body composition is important, especially if you aim for muscle gain, fat reduction, or merely fitness. Since peptides essentially speed up the muscle recovery process, help in repairing tissues, and enhance fat metabolism, this metric will directly reflect your progress.

II. **Blood Work and Hormonal Health:** Your blood tells a story about your health that goes beyond what you can see. A full blood panel gives insight into key biomarkers, such as hormone levels: testosterone, estrogen, cortisol, growth hormone, cholesterol, and inflammation markers (CRP), among many others. This becomes particularly important with peptide use since many peptides tend to affect hormonal balance.

Key biomarkers to track:

- **Testosterone and growth hormone:** These hormones play a very important role in muscle building, recovery, and the overall vitality of an individual. The CJC-1295 and Ipamorelin peptides amplify the natural levels of such hormones.

- **Thyroid function:** Your thyroid controls your metabolism. Peptides can help optimize this. Check for T3, T4, and TSH levels to make sure your metabolism is running as efficiently as it can.

- **Inflammation markers:** Chronic inflammation is going to hold you back, and peptides such as BPC-157 are great at reducing inflammation. Track markers such as C-reactive protein (CRP) to see how your inflammation improves.

Why It Matters: Understanding your hormone levels, along with other biomarkers, is crucial to getting the best results from your peptide regimen. You'll be able to adjust your peptide dosage along with other lifestyle factors to support hormone optimization, cellular regeneration, and overall vitality.

III. Vital signs and Cardiovascular Health: Baseline measurements of blood pressure, resting heart rate, and other indicators of cardiovascular health can provide a picture of how the heart is functioning before peptide therapy commences. Certain peptides, such as Thymosin Alpha-1, have been associated with immune-boosting properties and may offer benefits in terms of cardiovascular efficiency. These metrics are valuable to track.

- **Why it matters:** Overall, cardiovascular health is the very foundation of longevity. When your heart and circulatory system aren't working just right, peptides will help restore and support this very important system for a better health span and lifespan.

IV. Cognitive Function and Brain Health: Perhaps one of the most important benefits associated with peptide therapy is improved cognitive function.

Many peptides, such as Dihexa and Cerebrolysin, among others, support neurogenesis, memory, focus, and overall brain health. Consider cognitive assessments or tracking productivity and memory function before beginning peptide therapy.

- **Why it matters:** Most of us worry about cognitive decline as we get older. By measuring mental clarity, memory retention, and focus, you can monitor the improvement in brain function resulting from peptide therapy both in the short and long run.

V. Joint, Muscle, and Skin Health: Are you experiencing joint pain, muscle soreness, or skin issues at this time? You are to document all the physical discomfort that you might be experiencing since it will allow you to track the healing process assisted by peptides such as BPC-157 for joint and muscle recovery and GHK-Cu for skin rejuvenation.

- **Why it matters:** Peptides are great at encouraging tissue repair, collagen production, and inflammation reduction. In cases of physical injuries or discomfort, peptides hasten the healing process and return the functionality.

VI. Sleep and Recovery: Last but not least, monitor your sleep. CJC-1295 will increase deep sleep, which is extremely important for recovery, growth, and cognitive functioning. Sleep cycles, quantity of deep sleep, and overall sleep efficiency should be tracked through sleep-tracking apps or wearables.

- **Why it matters:** Sleep is the organic recuperation of the body.

Better sleep quality will ensure greater overall outcomes because peptides act much more effectively when your body is rested and in a highly recovered state.

By monitoring these important health metrics before beginning peptide therapy, you'll be able to track your progress and adjust your regimen to meet your goals to make sure you get the most out of your 60-day journey.

How to Find Safe and Reputable Sources for Your Peptides

Peptides should be sourced from safe and reputable suppliers. Many times, peptides are ordered online, and not all suppliers are created equally. It's best to know where to find legitimate sources to avoid buying counterfeit or low-quality products.

I. Research the Reputation of the Supplier: The first step in finding a reliable peptide supplier is researching the company's reputation. Reputable suppliers will generally receive positive feedback from customers and other professionals within the health and wellness community. Look for suppliers that have been around for several years and have built a decent reputation offering high-quality, research-grade peptides.

- **Features to watch out for include the following:** Credible reviews in forums and customer testimonials help a great deal in giving insight in the right direction. Suppliers with no or low online presence and those reported badly on many instances should be avoided.

II. **Third-Party Lab Testing:** Reputable peptide suppliers will also always provide third-party lab testing to ensure their products are pure and potent. Request certificates of analysis (COAs), which detail contaminant testing, purity, and concentration.

- **Why it matters:** Peptides are fragile compounds that have to be synthesized and stored correctly. Third-party lab testing ensures you get a pure, effective product without harmful additives or wrong dosages.

III. **Storage and Handling:** Peptides are generally required to be kept in cold conditions so that they may be effective. A given supplier should be in a position to provide peptides, handled, stored, and shipped in the best conditions. For instance, most peptides have to be shipped cold and must be accompanied by reconstitution instructions.

- **What to watch out for:** Vendors that provide cold-chain shipping - insulated packaging with cold packs - along with detailed instructions for storage and reconstitution of peptides can be more trusted.

IV. **Consult Healthcare Professionals:** Partnering with an experienced healthcare professional knowledgeable in peptide therapy will give you access to trusted suppliers. Many healthcare providers that utilize peptide protocols obtain their supplies from licensed pharmacies or pre-vetted suppliers.

V. **Avoid Unregulated Sources:** While their peptide vials might be much cheaper if one buys from unregulated companies, such firms usually offer low-quality, even dangerous merchandise. 32

You can only trust those organizations who follow legal directives and give proper information about sourcing.

- **Why it matters:** Poor-quality or counterfeit peptides waste your money and time. They can also be hazardous to your health.

VI. Know the Legal Status in Your Region: The legality of peptides varies in every country. In some regions, the peptides are just investigation compounds and are mostly prescribed or available only for research purposes. It is best to be informed about the legal requirements in your area as to the purchase of peptides to avoid any litigation.

Setting Your Health, Fitness, and Longevity Goals

The gateway to success with peptide therapy is setting clear and measurable goals. Whether the focus is anti-aging, muscle recovery, or cognitive enhancement, defined goals provide a way to track progress and stay motivated.

I. **Define Your Primary Objective:** Determine your main priority: Do you want to eliminate signs of aging, improve muscle strength, or increase cognitive function? Whatever your main priority is, that will determine your peptide protocol and all lifestyle changes you make within these 60 days.

- **Anti-Aging and Longevity:** If your primary focus is on anti-aging, peptides such as GHK-Cu and Thymosin Beta-4 will help improve skin elasticity, enhance collagen production, and help in cellular repair.

Set specific goals around improving the appearance of your skin, increasing energy levels, and feeling more overall youthful.

- **Muscle Growth/Recovery:** If your goals are focused on strength development and shortened recovery times, then peptides like IGF-1 and CJC-1295 should be of higher priority. You're going to want to set up your goals regarding an increase in lean muscle mass, a decrease in time for recovery between workouts, and an overall enhancement of physical performance.

- **Cognitive Improvement:** If the goal is to improve the activity of the brain, then some peptides do this, like Cerebrolysin and Dihexa, which help with focus, memory, and clarity. Examples of such goals could be improvements in productivity, enhancing memory retention, and the capability for better focusing on day-to-day activities.

II. **Set SMART Goals:** The SMART framework helps keep your goals actionable and trackable. Here is how to create a SMART goal:

- **Specific**: Explain exactly what you want to achieve.

- **Measurable:** Keep your goals measurable by using data.

- **Attainable:** Your goals should be attainable based on your current health and fitness levels.

- **Relevant:** Your goals should fall into place with your greater health and longevity goals.

- **Time-bound:** Set a timeline in which you would like to reach your goal within the 60-day period.

Instead of like, "I want to be healthier," here's a SMART goal: "I want to increase my muscle mass by 5%, and decrease my body fat by 3% in the next 60 days."

III. **Break Down Long-Term Goals into Short-Term Milestones**
Large goals can be daunting, so breaking them down into smaller milestones often makes them more manageable and helps motivate you. Consider dividing your 60-day journey into bi-weekly check-points:

- **By Week 2:** Improved energy levels, better sleep, and a noticeable increase in recovery speed.

- **By Week 4:** Visible improvements in skin elasticity, muscle tone, and cognitive clarity.

- **By Week 8**: Achieve the primary health objectives, including increased muscle mass, reduced inflammation, and improved cognitive function.

IV. **Monitoring Your Progress:** Write the daily and weekly progress in a journal, with any kind of fitness app, or even a tracking spreadsheet. Make regular measurements of such things as body composition, energy levels, the quality of sleep, and cognitive performance. Tracking the progress will keep you on track, plus you can make necessary tweaks to your regimen if needed.

V. Be Flexible: Peptide therapy is not one-size-fits-all, and you'll want to adjust goals or a stack of peptides as you go. You can find that some peptides work better for you than others, so be open to editing your protocol throughout the process when needed.

- **Example:** If you are building muscle at an incredible rate but aren't finding the energy levels you want, you may want to refine your protocol to include peptides such as Thymosin Alpha-1 for immune support and vitality.

VI. **Visualize Your Success:** Some of the most powerful techniques to help maintain motivation and stay on track are visualization exercises. Take some time each day to mentally rehearse - see yourself at the end of your 60-day journey after the health, fitness, and longevity improvements you set for your goal - and how great you are going to look, feel, and function after finishing your peptide regimen.

By setting clear goals and observing your progress, you will achieve everything you are after: not only the results but a meaningful, life-changing experience in peptide therapy.

Chapter 5

Weeks 1-2: Starting Strong with Peptide Integration

The first two weeks of your 60-day peptide therapy journey set the foundation for your success. You begin incorporating key peptides into your daily routine for anti-aging, vitality, and overall health enhancements. This chapter walks you through what to expect as you start your peptide regimen, begin making the necessary shifts in your nutrition to help support peptides, and incorporate some light exercise with recovery techniques.

Introduction to Your Peptide Regimen: Anti-Aging Focus

The first stage of your peptide administration is going to focus on the use of peptides that help in anti-aging and cellular regeneration. These peptides act at the deep cellular level to repair damaged tissues, enhance the production of collagen, and increase your body's natural healing processes.

I. **Peptides to Begin Treatment With:**

- **BPC-157: Although it will be a foundational peptide in your regimen, it is known for its powerful regenerative properties. It heals the gut lining; it repairs tissues and reduces inflammation. This is of much use to people with current injuries, digestive issues, or simply to recover faster after a workout.**

In addition, BPC-157 will also reduce oxidative stress and inflammation, two major drivers of aging, which will give it a notable set of anti-aging benefits.

- **GHK-Cu:** This is another copper peptide that should not miss a place in your anti-aging stack. It is mostly known for improving skin elasticity and getting rid of fine lines and wrinkles, increasing collagen production. More than this, GHK-Cu will help the body repair some tissues and regenerate at a cellular level, making it essential for aesthetic and health optimization purposes.

II. How to Use Them

The first two weeks are for the acclimatization of your body to these powerful compounds. Start with low to moderate dosages to minimize initial reactions and give your body time to acclimate.

- **BPC-157:** This is usually injected subcutaneously or taken orally. If injecting, inject around the area of injury/problem area for increased localized healing. If taken orally, on an empty stomach, this will optimize absorption for gut healing.

- **GHK-Cu:** is administered either topically for skin health or via injections to achieve more general anti-aging effects. Aesthetic benefits from the topical application of GHK-Cu can be visibly seen within two weeks.

III. Tracking Your Initial Results

A lot of the benefits from these peptides take time to appear, but you can start feeling subtle changes in skin texture, lessened inflammation, and higher energy levels within the first two weeks.

Document even the tiniest changes: digestion improvement, recovery times, and any positive changes on your skin. It will keep you motivated to further the program.

How to Adjust Your Diet for Optimal Results

When your body is nourished appropriately, the results of peptide therapy will be vastly improved. A clean, anti-inflammatory diet will allow peptides to work more effectively so you can achieve your goals of longevity, vitality, and anti-aging.

I. **Nutrient-Dense Foods**
Emphasis should be on whole, unprocessed foods rich in vitamins, minerals, and antioxidants that will help support cellular repair processes and lessen oxidative stress - one of the driving factors in the acceleration of the aging process. Nutritional intake during the first two weeks can be guided by the following specifications:

- **Lean Proteins:** Peptides stimulate the growth and repair of muscles, making appropriate protein intake important. High-quality sources include wild-caught fish, organic poultry, grass-fed beef, and plant-based proteins such as lentils or chickpeas.

- **Healthy Fats:** Peptides thrive on healthy fats - which also work to reduce inflammation and promote good brain health. Sources include avocado, olive oil, nuts and seeds, and fatty fish like salmon. These will also help with skin elasticity and hydration to give an added boost to the anti-aging effects of your peptide regimen.

- **Colorful Vegetables:** Fill your plate with a rainbow of vegetables high in antioxidants. Peptides such as GHK-Cu repair tissues and reduce oxidative damage; colorful vegetables - such as spinach, kale, carrots, and bell peppers - provide the antioxidants that power the process.

- **Bone Broth and Collagen:** Collagen will help the skin, joint functionality, and muscle recovery process. So far, bone broth is rich in collagen and amino acids, which will increase the impact of GHK-Cu and BPC-157 in giving you smoother skin and faster recovery times.

II. Decrease Intake of Inflammatory Foods

Inflammation is one of the biggest promoters of aging and degenerative conditions. Supporting your peptide therapy requires the removal or drastic reductions of inflammatory foods. Food to avoid include:

- **Refined sugars:** Sugar causes a spike in insulin, increases inflammation, and promotes aging through a process called glycation, which in turn causes a type of damage to collagen and elastin found in the skin.

- **Processed foods:** These are usually filled with bad fats, preservatives, and chemicals that create inflammation and nullify the benefits of peptides.

- **Too much alcohol:** It not only dehydrates the body, but it's also inflammatory. If you drink, let it be in moderate amounts of red wine, with its resveratrol - an ingredient linked with life extension.

III. **Supplements to Complement Peptide Action**

Aside from dietary changes, some supplements could further help your peptide regimen. They include:

- **Vitamin C:** This is crucial for collagen production and synergistic with GHK-Cu in facilitating skin and tissue repair.

- **Magnesium:** It plays a critical role in muscle recovery and cellular functions generally; hence, improving peptides' efficacy in dampening inflammation and relaxation.

- **Probiotics:** A healthy gut microbiome may help amplify the gut-healing actions of BPC-157. Adding a high-quality probiotic will give support for digestion and overall immune health.

Incorporating Light Exercises and Recovery Techniques

Exercise is the keystone in your 60-day journey, but the first two weeks should focus on gentle and consistent movement and recovery. Your body is already starting to begin the process of healing and repair via the peptides. Overtraining can slow down this process. Here's how to structure your physical activity in the initial phase:

I. **Low-Impact Cardio**

Light cardio exercises, like walking, swimming, or cycling, will increase blood flow to support your cardiovascular system and give you a great feeling, yet without putting your body under great stress.

Low-impact cardio should be done for 30 minutes 3-4 times a week for your body to adapt to the peptides and stimulate fat metabolism.

- **Benefits:** It optimizes blood flow, thus spreading peptides efficiently throughout your body. This also improves the heart condition for longevity.

II. **Yoga and Stretching**

Flexibility and stress reduction are generally neglected but are an integral component of any health program. The inclusion of yoga or stretching exercises into your routine will not only enhance your flexibility but also activate your parasympathetic nervous system in an effort to reduce stress and enhance sleep quality.

- **Why it matters:** Stress impairs healing and slows results. Light yoga or even mindfulness meditation can enhance the cognitive effects of peptides like Cerebrolysin but also contribute to your anti-aging goals by making sure cortisol levels remain low.

III. **Focus on Recovery**

The peptides that you are on during this period, like BPC-157 and GHK-Cu, work much better on a recovering body. Your body needs rest from the wear and tear of workouts. Give your body this period of rest; it's just as important as training. Make sure you're getting at least 7-8 hours of sleep per night and using other recovery techniques like:

- **Foam Rolling:** To release tension in muscles and improve blood flow.

- **Cold Therapy:** This can be done by taking cold showers or taking an ice bath. This will help reduce inflammation and speed up recovery.

- **Massage:** The deep tissue massages would further facilitate the process of recovery of muscles and thereby enhance the overall effectiveness of peptides such as BPC-157, which primarily promotes the healing of tissues.

III. **Tapered Increase in Intensity**

Within the first two weeks, your body gets accustomed to the peptides, as well as to the new routine. This is where you begin gentle increases in workout intensity for strength gains and endurance. The idea here is not to hurry but to allow the peptides to work in synergy with your body's natural recovery and growth processes.

These first two weeks of your 60-day journey are foundational in preparing your body for the profound changes the peptides will bring into it. Starting with low-dose peptides, adjustment of diet, and incorporation of light exercise while focusing on recovery - these are ways you set yourself up for success in the long term. Moving into the next phase, this progress you have made will accelerate, bringing you closer to your goals of longevity, vitality, and anti-aging transformation.

Chapter 6

Weeks 3-4: Enhancing Muscle Recovery and Cognitive Functions

As you approach the third and fourth weeks of the 60-Day Peptide Therapy Blueprint, now you are going to be ready for more advanced support for muscle recovery and cognitive function. This period in your peptide therapy is very crucial because you're going to add new peptides to target deeper muscle repair and enhance brain activity. You're also going to be refining your resistance exercises and your recovery techniques to optimize your results. Remember, stress management and optimization of sleeping patterns are also crucial in raising the efficacy of peptides.

Advanced Peptides for Repairing Muscles/Boosting Brains

In weeks 3-4, we are going to amplify the peptide protocol by adding in more advanced peptides that specifically target muscle repair and cognitive function. Your body should by now be responding well with the peptides from earlier in the week, and adding in new and more powerful peptides will only enhance your recovery process.

I. BPC-157: The Healing Powerhouse

BPC-157 is what's referred to as a regenerative peptide: used for accelerating healing in muscle, tendons, and ligaments. It not only fosters recovery after an injury but also facilitates the natural response of your body to resist the loss of muscle mass during high physical demand.

- **How it works:** BPC-157 is utilized for the regeneration of soft tissues and enhances the production of proteins required in soft tissues, such as collagen. This is partially achieved through its protective effects on cells which are important in the processes of healing and by inhibiting inflammation.

- **Benefits:** Faster recoveries from muscle strains and injuries, retaining more muscle mass, and increased tissue repair.

II. IGF-1 LR3: Supercharging Growth and Repair

IGF-1 LR3 is a long-chain recombinant of IGF-1, hence stimulating cell proliferation and replication, most especially in muscle cells. This increases protein synthesis, thus the body can recover faster from a workout, and it initiates the growth of lean muscle.

- **How it works:** IGF-1 LR3 increases the anabolic activity in the body, especially those processes concerned with the restoration of muscle mass after strenuous workouts. It increases cell division and repair due to its mimicking effects on growth hormones.

- **Benefits:** It speeds up muscle growth, increases muscle repair, and generally improves physical performance.

III. Cerebrolysin: A Brain-Boosting Peptide

Cerebrolysin is a peptide cocktail that can improve cognitive performance and promote brain health. During weeks 3-4, it becomes most beneficial, as mental clarity and focus are crucial for maintaining the right workout and recovery regime.

- **Mechanism of action:** Cerebrolysin stimulates neurogenesis (growth of neurons), improves memory, and enhances the general performance of the brain by protecting neurons from oxidative damage.

- **Benefits:** Enhanced concentration, improved memory, and learning capabilities, increased resistance against the stress on cognitive function.

With these sophisticated peptides added you will hugely improve muscle recovery and mental performance so your body and brain can stay in better shape as you forge ahead with your therapy.

Refining Your Exercise Routine for Maximum Muscle Recovery

With peptides that are more advanced to aid your recovery, this is the time to refine your workout to optimize muscle repair and avoid overtraining. The goal is to create a balance between intensity and recovery so you can build strength and endurance without putting additional strain on your muscles.

I. **Adjust for Recovery and Growth**
After weeks 1-2, you probably would have begun to feel much stronger, with toned muscles. Now you want to adjust the workouts to include more rest days or active recovery days-this is to allow time for the peptides to work effectively.

- **Suggested schedule:** You could alternate high-intensity workouts with lower-intensity swimming, walking, or yoga. This allows some rest for the muscles but still gives general movement and flexibility.

II. Progressive Overload

With peptides such as IGF-1 LR3 helping your muscles recover a bit faster, you safely can begin increasing the weights or resistance that you work out with. This idea is called progressive overload, which becomes necessary for further gains in strength.

- **Application:** Increase the weights you use by 5-10% on a weekly or bi-weekly basis, which would mean you are still maintaining proper form, and your recovery time is not compromised. Emphasize compound exercises to spur general muscular development; this includes squats, deadlifts, and bench presses.

III. Exercising Balance between Volume and Intensity

During all these weeks, it is about the balance between workout volume - the amount of work done totally - and the intensity, how difficult an exercise is. This way, you want to push your muscles to grow without getting injured or reaching burnout.

- **Suggestion**: Keep the workouts at around 60-75 minutes per week, mainly focusing on the intensity rather than the volume. Introduce compound lifts that hit more than one major muscle group; these are far more effective in overall muscle building. Combine intense workouts with recovery for a perfect balance to get maximum gains from your peptides.

.Stress Management and Sleep Optimization to Support Peptide Efficacy

Although peptides and workouts are important, at this stage of your journey, stress management and sleep optimization are really pivoting. A high level of stress and poor sleeping can offset peptide therapy and contribute to slower recovery and reduced cognitive performance.

I. **Cortisol Control:** Minimizing Stress for Optimal Outcomes Cortisol is a stress hormone that can inhibit the repair of muscles and promote fat deposition. In many individuals, high levels of cortisol impair cognitive functioning and interfere with clear focusing of the mind.

- **Mitigation of Stress:** Lowering cortisol levels through techniques such as meditation, breathing exercises, and yoga can greatly help in improving overall health. Even as little as 10-15 minutes a day of deep breathing or centering can greatly reduce stress and enhance the efficacy of peptides.

II. **Sleep: The Foundation of Recovery**
Sleep is where the magic happens - your body during deep sleep cycles goes into full repair mode. Growth hormone gets released, muscles get rebuilt, and your brain clears away toxins and regenerates neural pathways. Optimizing your sleep in weeks 3-4 supports the peptides you're using.

- **Sleep routine:** Get 7-9 hours of continuous sleep. It's very important to have a fixed sleep schedule and should develop a sleep-conducive wind-down routine, such as reading, light stretching, or listening to soothing music. Make sure to avoid screens for at least one hour before bed to help minimize the disruption of melatonin production due to blue light.

III. Supplements to Help with Sleep and Stress
Other aids that may help you in recovery could be magnesium, L-theanine, or ashwagandha; these make the level of stress minimal and enhance the quality of sleep. Magnesium relaxes your muscles, while ashwagandha regulates cortisol levels, bringing calmness and balance into your mind.

- **How to use:** Ingest the magnesium about 30 minutes before retiring to bed for a better muscle relaxation effect and deeper sleep. Ashwagandha can be taken in the morning or evening for better stress management and cognitive function.

The focus of weeks 3-4 in the 60-day peptide therapy blueprint is oriented toward making one's body robust, strong, resilient, and capable of performing optimally both mentally and physically. You will fully harness your therapy with the addition of advanced peptides, a re-fined exercise routine, and better optimization of stress and sleep management. Your muscles will recover at an accelerated rate, you will see improved cognitive function, and you will feel better and more energized than ever.

Chapter 7

Weeks 5-6: Longevity and Energy Maximization

Weeks 5-6 in the 60-Day Peptide Therapy Blueprint mark a poignant shift toward the core of long-term vitality and energy optimization. You are into the period in the journey where your body should have already started to yield positive changes in muscle recovery, cognitive function, and general well-being. Now it is time to expand those advantages with peptides specifically for longevity and extended vitality, along with changes in daily routine and the addition of intermittent fasting and supplements. This chapter will take you step by step on how to utilize peptides to maintain energy levels, revise your current exercise and recovery routines for success long into the future, and to combine peptides with both fasting and supplements for longevity.

Peptides for Extended Vitality and Energy Enhancement

The point at which you reach Weeks 5-6, the foundation for sustained improvements in physical and cognitive health has been laid. Now, attention shifts to using specific peptides that not only improve immediate performance but also promote long-term energy and longevity. These peptides will work at the level of enhancing mitochondrial function, regulating hormones, and enhancing general cellular health to help keep your body operating efficiently as you age.

I. Epitalon: The Longevity Peptide

Epitalon is among the strongest peptides, which has been

very well documented up to now for anti-aging and longevity. It controls melatonin production, supports telomere lengthening, and helps the organism to sustain its circadian rhythm-all the conditions necessary for a healthy life.

- **How It Works:** Epithalon works by increasing the production of telomerase, an enzyme protecting and elongating telomeres. Therefore, the length of telomeres is related to slower cellular aging and fewer cellular damages.

- **Benefits:** By regular application, Epitalon will favorably influence sleep improvement, DNA repair, or even the prevention of aging processes, giving you more energy and vitality as you progress through your peptide therapy journey.

II. **Motilin: Improvement of Metabolism and Gut Health**

Motilin is a peptide hormone in charge of controlling the functions of the digestive system. It ensures that digestion will be smooth, with effective absorption of nutrients, so that your body extracts from food everything it needs to keep the energy level high during the whole day.

- **How it works:** Primarily, motilin initiates stomach motility, thus allowing food to travel more smoothly in your body. Secondly, it aids in correct nutrient digestion for the proper absorption of all those desperately needed vitamins and minerals by your body for energy and vitality.

- **Positive Effects:** By keeping gut function in top

condition, motilin prevents bloating, fatigue, and energy crashes associated with improper digestion, which keeps you energetic and vital throughout the latter stages of your peptide regimen.

III. Thymosin Alpha-1: Immune Function

Thymosin Alpha-1 is a peptide famous for its immune-boosting action. During this phase, a healthy immune system helps you maintain your long-term energy and vitality. Chronic inflammation and infections excessively drain the resources that provide energy for you, whereas Thymosin Alpha-1, on the other hand, helps the body in fighting infections and reducing inflammation to result in an improved immune response of an individual.

- **How it works:** This peptide improves T-cell production, the most important constituent in adaptive immunity. The T-cells will enable your body to recognize and eliminate infected cells or cancerous cells. And improving such cells' production amplifies the capability of your body to maintain health and energy through the support offered by Thymosin Alpha-1.

- **Benefits:** Enhancing immune system activity, reducing inflammation, and increasing resistance to fatigue and illness are some points that will enable you to enjoy your vitality for an extended time.

How You Can Make Changes to Your Routine for Long-Term Success

During this period, your body has started to adapt to the peptide protocols that you have employed.

Now is the best time to dial in exercises, recovery, and peptide protocol for ongoing success and sustained energy. It's crucial to learn how to adapt each of these protocols according to how your body has reacted so far. This section of this chapter covers ways to listen to your body, make the necessary adjustments for longevity within your exercise routine, and maintain recovery properly.

I. Listening to Your Body

After many weeks of peptide therapy, you should have a much better idea about how your body reacts to both the peptides and adjustments in lifestyle. Take the time now to reflect on where you are seeing improvements and any setbacks, and make those changes in your routine as you go.

- **How to Adapt:** Keep a log of how your body feels throughout the day with regard to each peptide you take and any changes in exercise and foods. You can adjust the dosages as necessary, consult with a medical professional if you have an unexpected reaction, and adjust your exercise accordingly based on whether or not you feel energized or completely exhausted.

- **Why It Matters:** Your body is unique in its responses to peptide therapy, and understanding how you react will allow you to maximize the benefits and avoid negative effects. Sometimes, very subtle changes in your routine can yield long-term improvements.

II. Improving Your Exercise Routine

Here you will incorporate exercises to improve endurance and increase cardiovascular health, added to the muscle recovery.

Cardio and endurance training support heart health by improving stamina and maintaining consistent levels of energy throughout the day.

- **Exercise Modifications:** Add light to moderate aerobic exercise like swimming, cycling, or brisk walking to your regimen 3-4 times a week. Not only does this help your heart stay healthy, but it can also keep your mitochondria functioning at a high level, which will help keep energy levels up as you age.

- **Why It Matters:** Long-term vitality extends way beyond the realm of recuperation of muscles; it's about an all-rounded fitness approach. Cardiovascular health is closely associated with energy levels and longevity, and merging the latter with strength training may result in long-lasting benefits.

III. Enhancing Recovery

Recovery remains a big part of the process, even more so as you progress into the heavier peptides. Be sure to continue incorporating the recovery techniques that work best for you - yoga, meditation, or simply light stretching - into your routine.

- **Recovery Assistance:** You can also schedule active recovery days where you would be doing light movements and other methods, such as foam rolling, stretching, or massage. You can also include an infrared sauna or cold therapy equipment that would promote blood flow and reduce inflammation.

- **Benefits:** Better recovery optimizes your muscles and brain so that the peptides can work more effectively. Proper recovery also prevents injury and keeps the energy for the long term.

Combining Peptides with Intermittent Fasting and Supplements for Longevity

During Weeks 5-6, the peptide therapy can be further enhanced through intermittent fasting (IF) and supplements. These practices further support peptide efficacy, optimize metabolism, and assure general health and longevity.

I. Intermittent Fasting for Life Extension

Intermittent fasting is one of the most powerful ways to promote autophagy, a natural process in which the body cleans out damaged cells and generates healthy new ones. Combine intermittent fasting with peptides, and you will maximize the benefits of your therapy and drive longer-lasting vitality.

- **How to Begin:** The most popular method of intermittent fasting involves 16-hour fasts and an eight-hour eating window. This model allows one to create a natural time frame of not eating to promote fat-burning and cellular repair. In this model, your body will adapt to using fat for energy during the period of the fast, hence aiding in weight loss and longevity.

- **Why It Works:** Peptides including Epitalon and Thymosin Alpha-1 support intermittent fasting in cellular repair and immune function for further enhancing your effort in longevity and vitality.

I. **Supplementation to Improve Outcomes**

While peptides take center stage in your journey to health, supplements somehow complete the gaps and enhance their powers. There are certain supplements that work in harmony with peptides and improve mitochondrial function, reduce inflammation, and promote longevity.

Recommended Supplements:

- **NAD+ Boosters:** Nicotinamide Adenine Dinucleotide (NAD+) is a coenzyme essential in the process of energy production and cellular repair. Supplementation with Nicotinamide MonoNucleotide (NMN) or Nicotinamide Riboside (NR) will increase NAD+ levels to improve mitochondrial health and increase longevity.

- **Coenzyme Q10 (CoQ10):** An antioxidant that assists in energy generation at the cellular level through its optimizing effect on mitochondrial function, hence mitigating fatigue for a long and healthy life.

- **Resveratrol:** This powerful antioxidant, derived from red wine and grapes, promotes healthy aging through the activation of sirtuins-proteins responsible for modulating cellular health in response to and protection against age-related insults.

- **Why It Matters:** Peptides taken together with the right supplements can offer an integrated approach in longevity and energy optimization, catering to your body's needs and maintaining its health while aging.

III. Synergy Between Peptides and Fasting

This powerhouse of peptides combined with intermittent fasting optimally sets the stage for cellular repair, fat loss, and energy optimization. While fasting induces autophagy, peptides like **IGF-1 LR3** actually stimulate muscle regeneration, increasing your body's capability for creating and repairing tissues while concomitantly shedding fat reserves.

- **How it works:** Fasting cleans out the broken and damaged cells, while the peptides have the effect of growing new cells. This synergy between fasting and peptides enhances recovery, increases energy, and supports longevity. This dual approach also improves metabolic flexibility, allowing your body to shift between burning fat and carbs for fuel more efficiently.

- **Why It's Powerful:** If you use both fasting and peptides in your therapy, you will experience higher elevations in energy, fat loss, and vitality than either peptide or fasting therapy could produce alone.

Weeks 5-6 of the 60-Day Peptide Therapy Blueprint really creates a turning point in your health journey. By focusing on longevity, enhancing energy, and perfecting your routine, you set the right foundation to keep vitality going well into your future years. Intermittent fasting and other key supplements, including peptides designed to support cellular repair and enhance energy production, are going to significantly amplify your results. Make the proper adjustments, and you are going to find yourself well on your way toward unlocking health and longevity in a sustainable manner that ensures that.

Chapter 8

Weeks 7- 8: Finalizing Your 60-Day Transformation

Going through the final two weeks of the 60-Day Peptide Therapy Blueprint, most people find themselves experiencing a pretty noticeable difference in energy, cognitive sharpness, rate of muscle recovery, and overall health. These final weeks are all about cementing the progress that you have made, refining your approach for long-lasting results, and creating a plan for continued peptide use beyond the 60-day program. This will help you review the progress you have made, maintain the benefits you have achieved, and prepare for the next stage of your health optimization journey.

Reviewing Your Progress: Metrics and Health Improvements

It is important that in Weeks 7-8, one checks how far they have come. The last weeks of your peptide journey are all about reflection and decisions on the next steps you would take based on the success you were able to achieve. This section will walk you through how you can track your metrics, identify key improvements in your health, and places where you might still need to pay more attention.

I. Tracking Metrics

As we have identified throughout the program, some of the major metrics you need to focus on in gauging your progress will be:

- **Body Composition:** Monitor for changes in muscle mass, percentage body fat, and changes in overall body weight

- **Skin Health:** Evaluate for improvements in skin elasticity, skin texture, and general appearance including but not limited to youthful rejuvenation.

- **Cognitive Function:** Re-evaluate improvement in memory, focus, and clear-headedness.

- **Energy Levels:** Pay attention to everyday energy; if you have more energy during the day, and if your recovery is faster and easier post-workouts.

- **Quality of Sleep:** Note how rested you feel the next morning and if your sleep has improved both in length and depth.

II. Health Improvement Assessment

In the past fortnight, take the time to reflect upon how your health has improved across many different domains. Some questions to consider include, but aren't limited to:

- Is your skin looking younger and your muscles firmer?

- Are you feeling sharper mentally, more cognitively sharp?

- Are you recovering faster from workouts or physical activities?

- Are you sleeping better and more energized during the day?

These will be important to help make informed decisions about your continued use of peptides in relation to lifestyle changes that are needed to sustain and increase these results.

How to Maintain Youthful Skin, Muscle Strength, and Cognitive Health

Peptide therapy plays a huge role in maintaining youthful skin, strong muscles, and even cognitive capabilities. Beyond the 60-day program, it's essential to start making specific lifestyle changes that will support and extend the improvements you will have gained. The next steps outlined here will help you integrate peptides into a sustainable routine for long-term optimization of health. Whether glowing, radiant skin, resilient muscles, or sharp cognitive functioning - the rewards will keep on coming with just the right mix of habits and therapies.

I. Keeping the Skin Young

Perhaps one of the most visible benefits of peptide therapy is youthful, fresh skin. Peptides such as BPC-157 and GHK-Cu have played a very important role in the advancement of skin regeneration by boosting collagen production, facilitating the healing of tissues, and reducing inflammation. Going forward, the youthful appearance of your skin will be based on continued care, hydration, protection against environmental elements, and knowledgeable implementation of supportive therapies.

- **Hydration:** Perhaps the most easy and effectual skin-care strategies are those that involve staying hydrated. The skin starts to get older, it tends to lose moisture a little more easily, and can be prone to dryness and fine lines. Drinking at least 8-10 glasses of water per day will keep the skin elastic, promote cellular turnover, and help collagen production due to peptides. You can also use a humidifier if you happen to live in regions that are dry to avoid dehydration.

- **Diet for Skin Health:** Food intake in your body plays a vital role in how your skin looks and feels. Adding to your diet foods high in antioxidants such as berries, leafy greens, and nuts will help ward off free radicals-one of the leading causes of aging. Omega-3 fatty acids support skin elasticity and balance skin moisture, hence are essential for healthy skin, and can be sourced from foods like salmon and chia seeds. Most importantly, vitamins C and E are powerful antioxidants that promote the healing processes in compromised skin and also enable peptides to more effectively amplify collagen production. Take these vitamins through the intake of citrus fruits, nuts, seeds, and spinach to further enhance the anti-aging benefits of peptides.

- **Skin Care Routine:** The skincare regimen should further enhance skin renewal. Add to your products antioxidants, peptides, and hyaluronic acid, with its illustrious reputation for retaining moisture. Topical peptides, such as GHK-Cu creams, can be applied to enhance skin density, wrinkle reduction, and collagen production. Use serums or creams that contain peptides, which will help in continual repair and protection.

Cleansing, toning, moisturizing, and exfoliating all form part of a consistent routine in maintaining healthy, young skin.

- **Sun Protection:** The most crucial practice that keeps your skin young is protecting it from ultraviolet radiation. Certainly, peptides can be utilized to repair the damage brought about by the sun, but for sure, preventing further damage is always the starting point for long-term skin health. Apply broad-spectrum sunscreen with SPF 30 and above daily, even on cloudy days. Too much sun exposure can cause premature aging to lead to deep wrinkles, hyperpigmentation, and loss of elasticity in the skin. Wearing protective clothing and hats while going outdoors will give additional protection to your skin from harmful rays.

- **Collagen Boosting:** The peptide therapy encourages collagen production. However, it requires work to continue with high levels of collagen after the 60-day program. Adding this as a supplement to your routine, either in powder or capsule form, tends to be quite helpful. Collagen maintains skin structure, elasticity, and hydration - all of which are strong components of youthful-looking skin. Adding foods rich in vitamin C will enhance absorption and improve the effectiveness of collagen intake.

II. Sustaining Muscle Strength

The peptides taken during the 60-day program, particularly IGF-1 and CJC-1295, have greatly supported muscle recovery and growth.

Such peptides expedite the repair of tissues, reducing inflammation and boosting protein synthesis in tissues - important events in strengthening muscles and making them resilient. For the continuation or furtherance of gains, sustained attention to muscle maintenance becomes vital, through diet as well as the use of appropriate recovery techniques.

- **Strength Training:** Because peptide therapy works in concert with resistance exercises, namely weight training, the benefits also include building muscular mass and strength. To maintain the muscle mass and strength you have achieved, you need to continue your resistance training program at least 3-4 times a week. You should train all major muscle groups, including legs, chest, back, shoulders, and arms, and include compound exercises like squats, deadlifts, and bench presses, which work multiple muscles simultaneously.

- **Protein Intake:** Protein is an important nutrient for the repair and growth of muscles. To maintain the muscle strength one has built up while on a peptide regimen, it is necessary to keep a high level of intake of quality protein sources. Your daily protein need will vary based on your degree of activity, from 1.2 to 2.0 grams per kilogram of body weight. Lean meats, fish, eggs, quinoa other plant-based proteins, and whey protein are great sources. **This is especially true for post-workout nutrition. Consider adding a protein shake within a 30-minute window after your exercise to optimize recovery and muscle tissue building. Adding protein with carbs in that window will also help to restore muscle glycogen, further promoting recovery.**

- **Active Recovery:** Recovery is indispensable in the long-term maintenance and building of muscles. Keep adding active recovery techniques to your schedule each week, including yoga, light swimming, or even just stretching. These improve circulation and reduce muscle stiffness, thus improving flexibility and enhancing the recovery benefits of peptides. Massage and foam rolling also help your muscles recover by releasing tension in the fascia, which enables blood flow and reduces inflammation. By keeping your muscles pliable, you reduce tension in them, helping to maintain strength and prevent injury.

- **Supplementing for Muscle Health:** Continue with supplements such as Branched Chain Amino Acid (BCAA), creatine, and glutamine to help with the recovery and growth of the muscles. These work well with peptides to enhance synergy in reducing muscle breakdown, improving performance, and hastening up recovery times. Furthermore, magnesium supplements will help relax the muscles, preventing cramps and generally enhancing the muscles' function.

III. **Enhancing Cognitive Health:** Peptide therapy has given you great cognitive rewards by sharpening mental acuity, focus, and memory thanks to brain-boosting peptides like Cerebrolysin and Dihexa. You can, however, maintain this cognitive enhancement beyond the 60-day program by a combination of diet, mental stimulation, stress management, and support peptides.

- **Brain-Boosting Diet:** The human brain thrives on good food. The best way to keep and improve your brain health is by incorporating brain-boosting foods into your diet. Omega-3 fatty acids are essential to cognitive performance and can be found in foods such as fatty fish (wild-caught salmon), walnuts, and flaxseeds. These healthy fats support brain structure, promote neurogenesis - the creation of new neurons - and enhance mood and memory. Antioxidants from food, like berries, dark chocolate, and leafy greens, can protect the brain cells from oxidative stress, which is believed to be one of the major reasons for cognitive decline. In this way, regular consumption can slow down the aging process in the brain by preventing neurodegenerative diseases.

- **Mental Stimulation:** Just as the body requires exercise physically, so does the brain require it mentally. Engaging in mentally stimulating activities, such as working on puzzles, reading, or even learning new skills, keeps your brain active and sharp. Activities that keep your brain at work, like learning a new language or playing a musical instrument, stimulate neuroplasticity - that is, the brain's ability to adapt and reorganize itself. This is very important, especially in older age, for one who seeks to maintain as much cognitive function as possible. You can also try brain-training apps like Lumosity or Elevate, which will provide you with selected exercises for improving your memory, attention, and problem-solving skills, thus further enhancing your mental agility.

- **Stress Management:** Chronic stress has the ability to deplete the body and brain of energy, thus enabling cognitive decline, issues of memory, and mental fatigue. Stress levels can be significantly reduced with techniques designed to induce relaxation and clear the mind, such as mindfulness meditation, deep breathing exercises, and yoga. One can also reduce the risk of burnout and enhance cognitive functioning by incorporating short breaks into your schedule, particularly with mentally intensive work. Occasionally moving away from screens, taking a walk, or enjoying relaxation-type activities like journaling or listening to music may help keep stress at bay.

- **Sleep Optimization:** Sleep is an integral part of cognitive activity. While peptides, including Dihexa, do the repairs and protection on the brain cells, their power is really utilized when combined with adequate, quality sleep. It is during sleep that our brain sorts out information, fixes itself, and cements memories. Support brain health by sleeping 7-9 hours per night. Regularize your sleep schedule, reduce the amount of caffeine, and establish a relaxing bedtime routine to help improve sleep. Relaxation techniques, such as deep breathing or guided meditation, when done at bedtime, may decrease stress and improve sleep.

Planning for Continued Peptide Use Post-60 Days

While this 60-day blueprint has gone extremely well, it's time to talk about the future. Peptide therapy can and should extend beyond the initial 60 days to keep you healthy and vital.

This chapter will review how to incorporate peptides into your long-term therapy: how to cycle peptides when to take breaks, and how to integrate peptides with other therapies.

I. Cycling Peptides for Long-Term Use
Much like with any other type of therapy, peptide cycling will help avoid building up tolerance and give the body time to recover.

- **Peptide Cycling Protocol:** Upon completion of the 60-day program, one should then take a short break of 2-4 weeks before starting another round of therapy. This helps your body reset itself and retain its sensitivity to the peptides.

- **Rotational use of peptides:** You can also consider rotating different peptides based on your need and the benefit you want to achieve at a certain time. In one cycle you are on more cognitive-enhancing peptides while in the next, you are centered on peptides that improve muscle recovery or enhance longevity.

II. Combining **peptides with other therapies**
The outcome of peptide therapy will be much more effective once combined with other therapies and health-improvement lifestyle habits. This can be continued beyond the initial 60 days through the combination of peptide use with:

- **Hormone Replacement Therapy (HRT):** If your case involves an age-related deficiency of hormones, there's even more to benefit from when peptides are taken alongside HRT.

- **Supplements:** Continue boosting your peptide regimen with other supplements including NAD+ boosters, CoQ10, and antioxidants, for improved mitochondrial function and overall cellular health.

- **Diet and Exercise:** Peptides work even better when supplemented with a healthy lifestyle. Maintaining a healthy diet and exercise pattern will enable you to sustain the progress achieved through the use of peptide therapy for an extended period.

III. Creating a Long-Term Health Plan

Peptide therapy is a great tool for long-term optimization of health; however, it should be part of a larger plan. You may want to consider creating a personalized plan for your health which would include:

- **Periodic Health Assessments:** You will have to set up periodic visits with your physician to check on your progress, monitor vital indicators of your health, and alter your peptide medications as necessary.

- **Setting Goals:** Outside the 60-day mark, set new goals in terms of health and fitness that will keep you moving and on track.

- **Continuous Learning:** Stay updated with the most current information about peptides and health optimization. Science keeps evolving, and newer peptides or protocols may be available that can more profoundly affect your journey towards better health.

Weeks 7-8 mark the final stages of your 60-Day Peptide Therapy Blueprint, where you put it all together and will be creating a launch pad for continued success. The enhancement of vitality, cognitive functions, the recovery of muscles, and the improvement of general health could, through follow-up and long-term planning in using peptides, be even further than the initial 60 days. If strategically handled, peptide therapy will be at the very epicenter of your quest for a long-lasting journey to health, energy, and longevity.

Part 3:

Addressing Skepticism and Myths

Chapter 9

Debunking Myths About Peptide Therapy

Peptide therapy is one of the most exciting developments in modern health and longevity science, but it's often misconstrued. The misconceptions and myths about the safety and effectiveness of peptides have led some to consider the therapy with skepticism. Within this chapter, we're going to dig into and dispel some of the most common myths associated with peptide therapy, share scientific evidence supporting the use of peptide therapy, and explain why peptides are a safer alternative to traditional anti-aging and health optimization methods

Common Misconceptions About Peptide Safety and Effectiveness

Despite their ever-rising popularity, peptides are genuinely misunderstood and have created a number of myths surrounding their safety and effectiveness. Let's debunk some of the most common rumors and introduce some real facts that put things into perspective.

Myth 1: Peptides Are Steroids: Probably the most common rumor surrounding peptides is that they supposedly aren't any different from anabolic steroids. While peptides and steroids can both be taken for muscle growth and recovery, they actually possess some very distinct functional differences within the body. Steroids are lab-made hormones and have very severe side effects, such as liver damage, hormonal imbalances, and heart disease risks. Peptides are naturally occurring short chains of amino acids.

They heighten the body's processes, such as collagen or muscle repair. Because peptides tend to act in harmony with the body's natural functions, they are far less likely to cause the harmful side effects associated with steroids.

Myth 2: Peptides Are Unsafe and Unregulated: Another common myth is that peptides are unsafe because they are not regulated. In actual sense, while peptides are not as tightly regulated as pharmaceuticals; most of the peptides applied in therapies in countries that have strong health regulatory bodies go through stringent quality controls. In addition, the peptides employed in therapies are bioidentical to those present in the body, therefore diminishing adverse reactions. Peptides will be a safe, efficient treatment for a range of conditions, including anti-aging, muscle recovery, and cognitive enhancement when sourced from reputable vendors.

Myth 3: Peptide Therapy is for Bodybuilders: While peptide therapy is popular in the bodybuilding world due to its outstanding efficiency in muscle recovery and building, it is so much more than that. Medicine has increasingly been using peptides in such varied fields as anti-aging medicine, cognitive enhancement, immune system support, and more. Peptide therapy can help anyone wishing to enhance longevity, vitality, and good health, regardless of fitness level.

Myth 4: Peptides Are Not Scientifically Backed: Some have even said peptides lack scientific backing. This is no less than wrong. Scientists have been studying the actual effectiveness of peptides for many years, and many studies prove that they do make an impact in improving one's health.

Various other studies were dedicated to peptides such as BPC-157, which helps in repairing tissues, and GHK-Cu, which helps in skin regeneration. Other peptides, such as Thymosin Alpha-1, have been proven to enhance the immune system. Success with peptide therapy requires that one understands the type of peptides used and for what purpose.

Scientific Evidence Behind Peptides: Real-Life Case Studies

The thought of peptides was always shrouded in much doubt since not many people actually have any idea about the scientific evidence being used to prove their effects. While not every peptide has undergone quite the same amount of studies, many have shown amazing results in a clinical setting. In this section, we'll take a look at a few real-life case studies and the scientific research behind the powerful benefits of peptides.

I. BPC-157 for Muscle and Joint Repair: BPC-157 is actually an acronym for a peptide called Body Protection Compound. It happens to be one of the most researched peptides when it comes to helping with healing and tissue repair. Indeed, in several studies, BPC-157 has been shown to enhance the healing of muscles, tendons, ligaments, and even bone fractures. Clinical cases using BPC-157 included an athlete with a severe Achilles tendon tear. While conventional therapies never succeeded in completely curing the injury, upon the administration of BPC-157 into his rehabilitation program, the athlete went on to experience a rapid recovery, with full restoration of tendon function within weeks.

II. Anti-Aging and Skin Health with GHK-Cu: GHK-Cu is a very active copper peptide in the process of inducing skin repair and reducing the apparent features of aging. Clinical studies have proved that GHK-Cu peptide reduces fine lines, advances skin elasticity, and improves skin density. One of the most well-acknowledged studies involving GHK-Cu used a topical application of this peptide and documented a tremendous improvement in skin texture and firmness within a few weeks, thus illustrating its anti-aging molecule action.

III. Cognitive Enhancement with Cerebrolysin: Peptides are also under avid research for their cognitive enhancement properties. One of them is Cerebrolysin, a peptide derived from pig brain proteins that, in neurodegenerative disorders like Alzheimer's disease, has helped increase memory, concentration, and cognitive activity. It was noted during clinical trials with elderly patients that those suffering from cognitive decline had significant improvement in their memory and learning capabilities after months of administering Cerebrolysin.

IV. Thymosin Alpha-1 for Immune Health: Thymosin Alpha-1 is one of the peptides that has been in research for boosting one's immunity. Evidence has shown that Thymosin Alpha-1 can enhance the body's natural immune response, and because of that, it is very effective against infections and also enhances general immune health. In a patient with chronic fatigue syndrome, Thymosin Alpha-1 greatly improved energy levels and decreased the frequency of illness, overall enhancing immune function.

Why Peptides Are a Safer Alternative to Traditional Anti-Aging Solutions

Most anti-aging remedies involve the use of invasive treatments such as cosmetic surgery, Botox, and peeling chemicals. Though these treatments may improve appearance, which is temporary, they are accompanied by a significant level of risk like scarring, infection, and undesirable outcomes. Peptides offer a less hazardous, non-invasive alternative with long-lasting health and anti-aging benefits.

I. **Peptides Work in Harmony with Your Body, Not Against It:** One of the major positives of peptides has to do with their nature, which perfectly emulates the body processes. Unlike surgeries or artificial chemicals, peptides are naturally occurring in the body, controlling so many diverse vital functions such as tissue repair, collagen production, and hormone regulation. By enhancing these natural processes, peptides offer long-lasting improvements in health and appearance without many of the risks associated with more invasive treatments.

II. **Minimal Side Effects:** The conventional anti-aging treatments tend to have major side effects. For instance, botox can result in weakness in the muscles, drooping eyelids, and sometimes difficulty swallowing. Peptides have less adverse effects when applied excellently. Since they are bioidentical to your body's peptides, they are generally well-tolerated and have much fewer risks of adverse responses. Of course, peptides taken from reputed suppliers and in correct dosage are safer ways to achieve youthful, vibrant health.

III. Long-Lasting Benefits: Peptides work in the promotion of healing, regeneration, and cellular repair from inside out. This means that the benefits of peptide therapy can last long after the treatment period has ended. Unlike fillers or Botox, which only act temporarily, peptides treat the roots of aging and degeneration. In that respect, lasting improvements in skin health, muscle strength, and cognitive function are the reward. You can maintain youthful skin and tissue health for years to come using peptides such as BPC-157 or GHK-Cu, as opposed to continuous, expensive treatments.

IV Cost-Effective Solution: While most anti-aging therapies can be very expensive, peptide therapy tends to be moderately priced. Surgical procedures, fillers, and expensive skincare products cost upwards of thousands of dollars and often need to be continually updated. In contrast, peptide therapy offers long-term benefits at a fraction of the cost, making it accessible for anyone looking to optimize health and appearance without breaking the bank.

Over the years, peptide therapy has been riddled with myths and misunderstandings, but when the facts are clearly presented, it becomes clear that peptides actually represent a safe, effective, science-backed solution for health optimization and anti-aging. You will be able to understand the real science behind peptides and debunk common myths that will enable you to make a very informed decision about incorporating peptide therapy into your wellness routine. From increasing your energy to building muscle, improving cognitive function, and retaining youthful skin, peptide therapy offers a new paradigm for attaining long-lasting health and longevity.

Chapter 10

Safety Concerns and How to Use Peptides Responsibly

As peptide therapy gains momentum, it is not only its great possibilities one should become informed and excited about, but also its responsible use is something equally important. Peptides can offer potent health benefits with minimal risk when used appropriately, but at the same time, they require prudent management, just like any other therapy, to avoid adverse reactions. The important safety precautions to be considered in this chapter include avoiding sources of peptides that are not regulated, monitoring dosage and side effects, and cooperating with the health expert to ensure safety and effectiveness.

How to Avoid Unregulated or Dangerous Sources of Peptides

Perhaps the biggest problem with peptide therapy is the amount of unregulated, poor-quality peptide products available online. As peptides have grown increasingly popular, the market has become saturated with low-quality or even counterfeit products that can pose a serious risk to users.

I. The Dangers of Purchasing from Questionable Sources

The internet democratized access to peptides, but in turn, opened the door for numerous unregulated suppliers. More often than not, these suppliers sell peptides that are either impure or totally fake. Unregulated peptides can be stored improperly, adulterated with unknown chemicals, or mislabeled.

Such low-quality products, when injected, may result in dangerous consequences, such as contamination, infections, or even toxicity. In most cases, peptides purchased from non-reputable suppliers lack the purity they are supposed to have; this can be Peptides contaminated with harmful substances that your body may not be able to tolerate. These contaminants may cause immune responses or allergic reactions, at times very serious. Besides, peptides that are not stored well could deteriorate and hence become ineffective or even harmful.

II. How to Find Legitimate Sources of Peptides

If one wants to be protected, one needs to buy peptides only from recognized vendors that employ stringent quality control measures. Reputable and trusted vendors ensure their products comply with high standards by following Good Manufacturing Practices (GMP)-requirements. Compliance with GMP conditions is the way to ensure that peptide production corresponds to safety and quality checks at all levels of production. Reputable companies also provide certificates of analysis for their peptides, proof that they are pure and potent. The COA should be from an independent laboratory to confirm that the product is according to the advertised specifications. In addition, dependable peptide retailers have to store the peptides at appropriate temperatures, which in most cases require refrigeration, to maintain stability and effectiveness.

III. The Use of Third-Party Testing

Third-party testing is the surefire way to confirm a peptide product is safe.

Whenever you are purchasing peptides, the supplier should provide third-party lab test results for the sale. Tests need to confirm the identity of the peptide, its purity, and that it is free of any contaminants. Reputable suppliers will place these results on their website or provide them if asked. This is the level of transparency that will ensure the product you are using is safe and effective. Third-party testing ensures that someone other than the producer of the peptide is making sure the product meets or exceeds the stringent safety requirements, and thus, assures you a great deal. Vendors who cannot provide such documentation should be avoided since this is a surefire red flag that the product may not be as authentic or safe as it should be.

Managing Dosages, Cycling, and Potential Side Effects

While peptides on their own are generally innocuous, their administration must be very carefully controlled, observing recommended dosages, cycling them so that the body does not get used to them, and being highly cognizant of the possible side effects that might arise.

I. Determination of the Appropriate Dosage
Dosages of peptides are wide-ranging, depending on the type of peptide taken and the health goal to be achieved, as well as other variables such as age, body weight, and degree of general health. One of the most important parts of peptide therapy involves the right dosage; too little may not produce the desired effective result, while too much can lead to unnecessary side effects.

It means the dosage of growth hormone-releasing peptides, such as CJC-1295, has to be higher when targeting muscle gain and/or fat loss, whereas BPC-157 needs only a small dose in tissue repair. It is always safer to start with a dose that is low enough but likely to work and then go up gradually, giving your body the time to respond. This may be done with the help of your medical professional, who would pay attention to the dosing so that you tailor the dosage in a way that you achieve the very desired results without crossing the line into the harmful zone.

II. Peptide Cycling for Maximum Benefits

Cycling peptides refers to their administration over a period of time - usually 4 to 6 weeks - followed by cessation of use for several weeks before recommencing. Cycling the peptides is of paramount importance, as continuous administration would lead to desensitization in which your body becomes less responsive over a period of time. By properly cycling, you are allowing the body to reset its peptide receptors for maximum efficiency of the therapy. Besides, cycling minimizes risks for possible long-term side effects from overuse. Peptides that increase IGF-1, such as CJC-1295, must be cycled in order not to get excessive levels of IGF-1, which could trigger unwanted growths or metabolic disturbances.

III. Being Aware of Possible Side Effects and How to Manage Them

The peptide therapy is usually well-tolerated, and it may have a minimal risk for side effects when administered appropriately.

Minor problems that many may have include injection site reactions - redness, swelling, or itching. Other possible side effects might be headaches, dizziness, or nausea if the dosages are too high and peptides are not cycled properly.

Of course, in rare cases, peptides influencing an increase in the level of some hormones-for example, IGF-1-may have serious side effects that may include excessive water retention, joint pains, or hormonal imbalances. The early recognition of such signs and dosage adjustment or temporary cessation may avoid further complications.

It is also very important to use the proper protocols with the injections, like using sterile needles and rotating injection sites to avoid tissue damage or infection. Monitoring one's body response and being aware of changes will be key to safe and effective peptide use.

Professional Health Monitoring of Peptide Therapy

Peptide therapy, for safety and efficacy, should be performed under the auspices of a qualified healthcare professional. Peptide self-administration based on information read from the internet or here and there is not devoid of risks, as the body of everyone reacts differently to these compounds.

I. The Need for Medical Supervision
It is always a good idea, however, to consult with a healthcare professional who has experience with peptide therapy to get advice that is particular to your needs and goals.

To begin, they assess your general health through blood tests and your case history to determine if this type of peptide therapy will work for you.

Once initiated, your physician will be able to evaluate the response, titrate dosages, and manage potential side effects. They are thus in a good position to be able to offer complementary therapies that enhance the efficacy of peptides by either nutritional adjustments or other therapies. They can have regular follow-ups to ensure the therapy is functioning without any unforeseen setbacks in health.

II. Lab Testing and Monitoring

One of the most integral parts of medically supervised peptide therapy involves regular lab testing. In other words, blood tests are going to keep track of key markers such as IGF-1 levels, liver function, and kidney health. Observing these markers averts long-term potential risks that may include over-stimulation of growth factors, which can be very detrimental to health in the form of cancer or organ stress.

Regular health checks will also allow your medical professional to adjust peptide dosages based on real-world data. If, for example, blood tests show that IGF-1 is too high or your liver is stressed, your physician might ask you to lower the dosage of peptides or cycle them off for a while.

III. Tailored Treatment Regimens

Everyone's body is different in how it reacts to peptide therapy, and for this reason, a health professional will be helping to tailor your program to your needs and goals.

Be it muscle recovery, cognitive enhancement, or anti-aging, your doctor will select the right combination of peptides while adjusting dosages and modeling a long-term approach that ensures safety and sustainability.

It will also make sure that you are taking peptides more safely and effectively. Moreover, the physician will be able to instruct you through changes in other life aspects that might be impacting peptide therapy, which includes but is not limited to your diet, exercise routine, and sleep habits.

IV. Diagnosis and Management of Side Effects

Medical follow-up is extremely important in managing all kinds of side effects. Mild side effects, at times, can be easily corrected through adjustment in dosage or changing the peptide being administered. However, more serious side effects may require cessation of the therapy. A healthcare provider can help verify when it will be safe to continue or when it is best to discontinue peptides.

Part 4:

Lifestyle Strategies to Maximize Peptide Effectiveness

Chapter 11

Nutrition for Longevity and Recovery

Peptide therapy, which is probably one of the most effective tools for longevity, vitality, cognitive function, muscle recovery, and overall health, will be brought to a whole new level with strategic dietary choices. Just as peptides work at the cellular level in the body to repair, regenerate, and optimize, nutrition provides the foundational support needed to amplify these effects. This chapter explores nutrition and how it plays a critical role in complementing peptide therapy, showing dietary strategies that can be put into place to optimize the benefits of your 60-day peptide regimen and beyond.

The Role of Diet in Enhancing Peptide Results

With proper nutritional support, peptides can exert their full potential in the body for healing, repair, muscle building, enhancement of cognition, and anti-aging. Through nutrition comes the substrates, amino acids, antioxidants, vitamins, and minerals that provide a conducive environment for peptides to work optimally.

I. Feeding Cellular Repair and Regeneration

Tissue repair and regeneration are mediated by peptides such as BPC-157 and Thymosin Beta-4. These, however, need an adequate availability of nutrition to help in cellular turnover for healing. Amino acids are the subunits of proteins that are highly needed in the recovery of muscles and repair of skin.

Ensuring your diet is full of high-quality proteins-like lean meats, fish, eggs, and plant-based proteins such as legumes and quinoa-can help accelerate the recovery processes induced by peptides.

The general intake of vitamins and minerals, including Vitamin C, zinc, and magnesium, is crucial for collagen synthesis, immunity, and cellular replication. Without these nutrient levels, the optimum advantages of peptide therapy may not be fully utilized by your body, and this might impede visible results.

II. Minimizing Inflammation to Support Peptide Function
Long-term inflammation harms the body's self-repair processes and reduces its response to peptide administration. Several peptides have anti-inflammatory properties, such as GHK-Cu and BPC-157, and promote repair, but this will be grossly enhanced when there is an absence of pro-inflammatory components in the diet. When you consume foods high in antioxidants (such as berries, leafy greens, and nuts) and omega-3 fatty acids (found in fish, flaxseeds, and walnuts), along with other anti-inflammatory compounds, you are creating an internal environment that supports the action of peptides. Such nutrients ease oxidative stress, improve cell function, and increase the general health

On the other hand, foods that create inflammation, such as processed sugars, refined grains, and trans fats, should be avoided to maximize peptide effectiveness. These harmful foods can activate inflammatory pathways that act against the healing benefits brought about by peptides; thus, this will make their recovery and aging processes even slower.

III. Hydration and Peptide Efficacy

Hydration is one of the most important factors in ensuring peptides are well circulated through the bloodstream, reaching their target cells. Cellular function will be hampered by dehydration, impeding the processes in which peptides may have a role to play in tissue repair, skin regeneration, or muscle recovery. To maintain optimum functionality of peptides, drink at least eight glasses of water a day and more if you are into highly strenuous exercise or living in hot climates.

Proper hydration, on the other hand, helps with detoxification, which means to cleanse the body from all waste products and toxins that may interfere with the proper absorption of peptides, hence helping in maintaining healthy cells. A well-hydrated body automatically reflects clear skin, proper digestion, and agile cognitive function - all areas that peptide therapy seeks to improve.

Superfoods, Supplements, and Anti-Inflammatory Diet Choices

Nutrition doesn't stop at just simple macronutrients: proteins, carbohydrates, and fats. Superfoods and certain supplements guarantee a further increase in health, synergistically working with peptides.

I. Superfoods for Improved Peptide

Superfoods are foods characterized by high nutrient value and can provide great health benefits because of the high content of vitamins, minerals, and antioxidants.

The inclusion of such products into the diet may complement the treatment with peptides because of the improvement of recovery, decrease of oxidative stress, and support of general health.

Some of the most helpful superfoods taken together with peptides include:

- **Berries:** Blueberries, Raspberries, Blackberries. They contain loads of antioxidants that help fight against oxidative stress and inflammation.

- **Leafy Greens:** Spinach, kale, Swiss chard - all of these host a great deal of vitamins A, C, and K, which are really good for collagen synthesis, among other functions of the cells.

- **Nuts and Seeds:** Almonds, chia seeds, and flaxseed provide healthy fats, especially omega-3s, that reduce inflammation and promote brain health.

- **Fatty Fish:** Salmon, mackerel, and sardines are healthy sources of omega-3 fatty acids for reducing inflammation, aiding in the recovery of musculature, and sharpening cognitive functions.

- **Turmeric:** This superfood has a powerful anti-inflammatory compound called curcumin, which can be helpful in quicker recoveries from injuries and reducing the chance of chronic diseases.

II. Supplements to Complement Peptide Treatment
While a well-rounded diet meets the majority of nutritional needs within the body, supplements complement the deficiencies and enhance the efficacy of peptide therapy.

- **Collagen Supplements:** Most peptides have something to do with regenerating your tissues and skin. Consequently, supplementing with collagen peptides amplifies the elasticity of the skin, minimizes fine lines and wrinkles, and aids in maintaining healthy joints. Collagen supplements provide the raw materials for the body's natural repair processes.

- **Omega-3 Fatty Acids (Fish Oil or Algal Oil):** These are anti-inflammatory supplements and have a supporting effect on cognitive health; thus, they act very well in support of the nootropics peptides such as Cerebrolysin and Dihexa.

- **Vitamin D**: Since it is considered very vital for immune function, the health of the bones, and overall vitality, Vitamin D can support peptides that help improve physical and cognitive performance.

- **Magnesium:** This mineral is highly essential in the relaxation of muscles, quality sleep, and stress management; its role becomes particularly important when combined with peptides for recovery and cognitive enhancement.

III. Anti-Inflammatory Diet Choices

Following an anti-inflammatory diet is important to make sure peptide therapy works at its best. Such a diet aims at reducing foods causing inflammation and leading to oxidative stress, joint pain, and poor cellular health.

The major components of an anti-inflammatory diet include:

- **Whole Grains:** brown rice, quinoa, oats. These are high in fiber and regulate blood sugar well, helping to avoid insulin spikes and subsequently lowering inflammation.

- **Healthy Fats:** Avocados, olive oil, nuts. These are rich in monounsaturated fatty acids that reduce inflammation and enhance the activity of the brain.

- **Lean Proteins:** chicken, turkey, beans. Lean sources of protein provide all the essential amino acids without the inflammatory effects of processed meats.

- **Cruciferous vegetables: like broccoli, cauliflower, and Brussels sprouts,** are wonderful foods, rich in antioxidants and fiber, which help cleanse the system of impurities and reduce inflammation.

Avoid inflammatory triggers such as:

- **Processed Sugars:** These spike blood sugar levels and trigger inflammation.

- **Refined grains - white bread and pasta** - these are grains devoid of fiber that can cause spikes in blood sugar, leading to inflammation.

- **Trans Fats:** Fried foods, baked goods, and a few margarines serve as carriers of trans fats, which lead to chronic inflammation and cardiovascular ailments.

By following the anti-inflammatory diet, you are creating an optimal internal environment in which the peptides work to reduce inflammation and promote quicker, more effective recovery.

Personalized Diet Plans for Different Peptide Protocols

Not all peptide protocols are the same, and the nutritional needs will also differ depending upon the type of peptides taken. Whether one is focused on muscle recovery, improving cognitive function, or even anti-aging, one can ensure super-charged results once the diet is tailored to that peptide regimen.

I. Muscle Recovery and Performance

If recovery and muscle performance are your main focuses, IGF-1, CJC-1295, and BPC-157 will be at the forefront of your protocol. While all three aid in muscle growth, repair, and recovery, they ultimately depend on a diet high in protein to work their magic.

Centre your diet around high-quality protein sources, such as:

- **Lean Meats and Fish (Chicken, Turkey, Salmon):** These are necessary for rebuilding muscle tissue.

- **Plant-Based Proteins:** quinoa, lentils, beans-all great sources of complete amino acid profiles and help in muscle repair and total body health.

- **Whey or Plant-Based Protein Powder:** This is great post-workout for ensuring you get enough protein to support recovery.

II. Cognitive Enhancement and Brain Health

For peptides like Dihexa, Cerebrolysin, and Semax with cognitive enhancement properties, one should adopt a brain-boosting diet that includes plenty of omega-3s, antioxidants, and other nutrients protective of the brain. Key dietary focuses include:

- **Omega-3s and Fatty Fish:** Fatty fish, like salmon, contains DHA, a critical building block of brain cell membranes, which is highly important to the health of the brain.

- **Antioxidant-Rich Foods:** Berries and dark chocolate reduce oxidative stress in the brain, enhancing memory and cognitive function.

- **Nuts and Seeds:** These are rich in vitamin E; several studies have proven that it prevents cognitive decline.

III. Anti-Aging and Skin Health

GHK-Cu and Thymosin Beta-4 are generally administered for skin health and anti-aging, helping reduce wrinkles, improving collagen production, and enhancing elasticity. Support these peptides with foods that improve collagen production and foods rich in antioxidants.

- **Collagen Rich Foods:** The most crucial here would be bone broth and chicken skin, which give the building blocks necessary to create collagen.

- **Foods High in Vitamin C:** These foods include citrus fruits and bell peppers; vitamin C really plays a massive role in collagen creation and skin health.

- **Foods that Hydrate:** These are cucumbers and watermelon. Hydrating helps to keep the elasticity in the skin and aids in preventing it from aging prematurely.

Chapter 12

The Importance of Sleep and Stress Management

Sleep and stress management are major components of peptide therapy to optimize one's health. Without proper sleep and stress management, peptides have very limited effectiveness, despite the spectacular benefits they provide in areas of muscle recovery, cognitive function, and anti-aging. This chapter goes into significant detail on how sleep and stress affect peptide therapy and provides you with some very real tangible techniques you can use to maximize your 60-day peptide journey and well beyond.

How Sleep Enhances Peptide Efficacy for Muscle Repair and Cognitive Health

Arguably one of the most crucially important, yet least considered, factors in overall health - and especially in terms of peptide therapy - is sleep. Deep sleep cycles are when most of the recovery and repair processes take place in your body. Peptides like IGF-1 and BPC-157 work with your body's self-healing mechanisms to regenerate muscle tissue, enhance cognitive function, and repair damaged cells, if your body is in a restorative state, which sleep provides.

I. Muscle Recovery and Growth During Sleep

While the role of peptides in recovery processes for muscles cannot be overemphasized, these effects are heightened during sleep. Muscles are microtorn each day from physical activities and exercise; these need to be recovered.

Peptides taken to spur this, including IGF-1 (Insulin-like Growth Factor-1) and CJC-1295, would see the bulk of their repairing mechanism occur in deeper stages of sleep.

- **Growth Hormone Release:** Growth hormone release, responsible for muscle growth as well as tissue repair, occurs at its peak during deep sleep. Peptides like CJC-1295 stimulate this release and, in turn, help in better muscle recovery. Sleepless nights or less sleep results in low GH levels, which diminish the effect of peptides responsible for muscle repair.

- **Protein Synthesis:** Muscle repairs require the synthesis of protein, which occurs most actively while an individual sleeps. Good sleep will ensure that the peptides you are using can increase the rate of protein synthesis and hence growth and strength of muscles. On the contrary, the limitation of sleep will partly inhibit this important process, hence slowing down recovery times and reducing gains from exercising.

II. Sleep and Cognitive Function

The actions of peptides, such as Cerebrolysin and Dihexa, are to enhance cognitive function: memory, focus, clarity of mind. However, their effects are modulated by the quality of sleep. Sleep is a method used by the brain to consolidate memories, repair neurons, and clear out toxins, processes that peptides amplify.

- **Memory Consolidation:** Sleep is an important aspect of memory consolidation, wherein information is processed and stored for future use.

Cognition-enhancing peptides can only optimally function if time is given to solidify new neural connections within the brain during sleep.

- **Neuroplasticity:** Dihexa and other peptides promote neuroplasticity, or the ability of the brain to form and reorganize synaptic connections. Deep sleep is one critical period where neuroplasticity takes place, whereby the brain cells update themselves after new learning and experiences. Sleep deprivation slows the neuroplastic changes and can negate the brain-enhancing activity of peptides.

- **Waste Removal:** Sleep turns on the glymphatic system, which cleans metabolic waste from the brain. This process is enhanced by peptides that are designed for brain health. Poor sleep disrupts waste removal and leads to cognitive fog, poor memory, and decreased mental sharpness.

III. Optimizing Sleep for Peptide Results
High-quality sleep should be prioritized to maximize peptide therapy benefits. Among the key strategies are the following:

- **Stick to a Sleep Schedule:** Go to bed and wake up at the same time each day. This will help your body maintain its natural rhythm, allowing it to work properly and optimize sleep quality.

- **Create a Calming Bedtime Routine:** Engage in relaxing activities before bedtime, such as reading, meditation, or light stretching, to help tell your body it's time for sleep.

- **Limit Exposure to Blue Light:** The blue light of phones, tablets, and computers inhibits the production of melatonin, a sleep-regulating hormone. For one hour before bedtime, avoid the screen.

- **Perfect your sleep environment:** Ensure the bedroom is cold, dark, and quiet. Blackout curtains or a white noise machine will help if necessary.

Practical Stress Reduction Techniques to Support Overall Well-Being

While peptide therapy can work wonders for both body and mind, stress can very well sabotage your results. Chronic stress is indeed a well-documented inhibitor of many physiological processes, including those that peptides aid. High levels of stress raise cortisol - a hormone known to interfere with peptide efficacy by slowing recovery, increasing inflammation, and reducing cognitive function. Learning how to handle or manage stress effectively helps support the overall benefits of peptides.

I. How Stress Affects Peptide Therapy

The peptides you are administering to stimulate muscle recovery, anti-aging, and cognitive function essentially serve to amplify your body's own natural processes. The problem is that chronic stress can directly negate many of these.

- **Cortisol and Muscle Recovery:** The more cortisol within one's body, the more muscle breakdown, the slower the recovery time, which in turn decreases the effectiveness of peptides for muscle-building, such as IGF-1.

Cortisol is catabolic; it degrades proteins and prevents the creation of new muscle tissue.

- **Cognitive Decline:** Chronic stress causes neuron damage and deteriorates memory and learning, therefore nullifying the overall improvement that peptides like Cerebrolysin might induce in cognition. More precisely, high cortisol levels have been associated with reduced hippocampus volumes - a brain region responsible for memory and learning.

- **Inflammation and Aging:** Stress acts as a stimulant of pro-inflammatory processes that cause cellular aging and reduces the anti-inflammatory activity of peptides like BPC-157. More inflammation may accentuate certain features of aging, coupled with poorer wound healing and an overall decline in health.

II. Practical Stress Reduction Techniques

Stress management plays a significant role in maximizing peptide therapy. Reducing stress with simple daily activities will lower cortisol levels and enhance recovery, boosting overall well-being. Here are some practical techniques that will help you manage stress:

- **Mindfulness meditation:** it has been shown to reduce cortisol levels, enhance mood, and sharpen mental clarity. As little as 10 to 15 minutes of meditation daily may greatly reduce the levels of stress and enhance one's ability to focus.

- **Deep Breathing Exercises:** Deep, slow breathing activates the body's relaxation response, slowing the heartbeat, lowering blood pressure, and quieting the nervous system. Diaphragmatic breathing techniques or the 4-7-8 breathing method can keep acute stress in check all day.

- **Physical activity:** Many general benefits of exercise as a stress-reducing technique are well-documented. Exercise tends to stimulate the release of endorphins, or the body's natural mood elevator, promoting sleep in general. Of course, intense workouts should be equally balanced with rest and recovery, especially while on a peptide regimen, to avoid overtraining.

- **Yoga and Tai Chi:** are good for stress reduction, flexibility, and mindfulness. It tends to regulate the nervous system and evokes calm; hence, it is a very good combination with peptide therapy.

- **Journaling:** Putting your thoughts and feelings on paper is a very powerful means of managing your stress. Journaling helps to put things into perspective, deal with your feelings, and unload judgments that may be affecting your mental and physical health.

- **Social Links:** Efforts at engaging a supportive community or spending time with friends and family can reduce levels of stress and improve emotional well-being. Social connections trigger the release of oxytocin, which is a hormone that works against cortisol, promoting relaxation and happiness.

- **Nature Exposure:** Spending time outdoors, especially in green spaces, has been shown to cut down stress and improve mood. Whether it's taking a walk in the park or a weekend hiking trip, there is connectivity with nature that works in lowering stress levels.

III. Balancing Work and Life to Reduce Stress

Work is where most people get their primary stress from. A healthy balance between work and personal life can eliminate much of the stress and keep overall well-being intact. The following are a few tips to bring about better work-life balance:

- **Setting boundaries:** Clearly distinguish between work time and personal time. This may involve abstaining from checking emails or working late at night to avoid interfering with sleep and increasing stress.

- **Prioritize Tasks:** Stress more on finishing the high-priority work and never hesitate to hand over any responsibilities or say no to them in case of being burdened.

- **Take Breaks:** Take regular breaks throughout the day. This will help recharge from the inside out and thus prevent any kind of burnout. Even small walks or deep breathing for a few minutes reduce stress and enhance focus.

Some of the most important factors that will play a huge role in the effectiveness of your peptide therapy involve lifestyle factors, including sleep and stress management. You help create an internal environment that supports muscle recovery, cognitive health, and overall vitality by making quality sleep a top priority and developing functional methods to reduce stress. This would include designating some lifestyle approaches that will complement the beneficial effects of peptides; hence, it will promote long-term health.

Chapter 13

Exercise Plans Tailored to Peptide Therapy

Exercise plays an important role in any program geared toward health optimization; peptide therapy really turbocharges it for better longevity, recovery of muscles, cognitive health, and vitality. IGF-1, CJC-1295, BPC-157, and Thymosin Beta-4 are some of the peptides contributing to this by enhancing muscle repair, improving endurance, and shortening recovery times, hence allowing higher levels of physical stresses that yield much better results. However, to fully exploit these benefits, one must engage in a certain form of exercise regimen, which will complement peptide treatment. This chapter considers how strength training, cardiovascular workouts, and mobility exercises can be specifically tailored for those undergoing peptide therapy and how to maintain these habits post-therapy.

Strength Training and Cardio for Optimal Recovery

While both strength training and cardiovascular exercise form the backbone of any good fitness program, they also become even more effective with the introduction of peptide therapy. IGF-1 and CJC-1295 peptides support the creation of lean body mass through the growth of muscles and tissues and fat metabolism. These make them perfect for anyone who is after lean muscle development while improving cardiovascular health. Here's how to tailor these workouts to align with your peptide protocol.

I. Strength Training: Maximizing Muscle Growth and Recovery

Strength or resistance training is essential for building lean body mass, enriching bone density, and boosting general body strength. It finds its complement in such peptides as IGF-1, which boosts cell proliferation and muscle growth. To fully exploit the potential of your peptides, apply the following principles:

- **Compound Exercises:** Focus on compound exercises targeting a group of muscles, such as squats, deadlifts, bench presses, and pull-ups. This will not only be able to stimulate more muscles but also trigger your body to release growth hormone, whose activity is further enhanced by peptides like CJC-1295. Throw peptides into the mix, and your recovery period speeds up so you will be able to train well without being bothered about overtraining.

- **Progressive Overload:** One cannot just continue training with the same weight repeatedly and expect to see progressive muscle gain. Progressive overloading of muscles does stimulate tissue repair and its hypertrophy. This is further enhanced by peptides like BPC-157, which help reduce inflammation and speed up recovery.

- **Rest Between Sets:** While peptides speed up recovery, appropriate rest between sets is paramount to allow muscles time to rebuild energy and repair. Normally, one is advised to take 1-3 minutes rest between every set of exercise, depending on your workout intensity.

- **Recovery Days:** While peptide therapy decreases muscle soreness and speeds up recovery, your body does require some rest time. Incorporate at least 1-2 recovery days in a week to avoid getting burned out and overtraining while peptides do their magic job in the background.

II. Cardiovascular Exercise: Enhance Endurance-Burn Fat

Cardio contributes to heart health, increases endurance, and will contribute to fat loss. Therefore, peptides can be utilized for increasing metabolism and enhancing endurance so that one can do longer cardiovascular exercises without getting tired. Peptide therapy with cardio will contribute to increased overall fitness and enhance your strength training.

- **Interval Training:** High-Intensity Interval Training (HIIT) is the most effective form of cardio that accompanies peptide treatments. It consists of short lengths of high-intensity exercise followed by rest. This method activates fat burning, especially when peptides supporting fat metabolism, like AOD9604, are involved, and also builds cardiovascular endurance.

- **Steady-State Cardio:** Such as jogging, cycling, or swimming at a moderate pace to improve your heart health and stamina. This will help improve your aerobic capacity without putting your body under too much stress. The peptides will help you recover quicker in between sessions, which means you can do more cardio without risking injury.

- **Peptides and Fat Loss:** The peptides CJC-1295 and Ipamorelin trigger fat metabolism by initiating the secretion of growth hormones. In addition to this, cardio exercises that increase the heart rate and maintain it for 20-30 minutes, a few times a week, will maximize fat loss.

Exercises to Maximize Longevity and Mobility

Longevity is more than just aging; it's remaining mobile, strong, and intellectually active during the course of one's life. Peptide therapy helps a person to feel younger with quicker recovery, lean muscle mass, and healthy joints and tendons. However, some forms of exercise that will build flexibility, mobility, and functional strength are vital for maintaining long-term physical health.

I. Mobility and Flexibility: Prevention of Injury and Allowance of Continued Range of Motion
Mobility exercises help maintain or preserve the range of motion within your joints and muscles, which is very important for injury prevention, especially as you get older. Peptides such as Thymosin Beta-4 encourage joints, tendons, and ligaments to heal, making mobility exercises even more valuable.

- **Dynamic Stretching:** The inclusion of dynamic stretching before any type of exercise gears up the muscles and joints to function and, as a result, prevents the chances of injury. These are the movements such as leg swings, arm circles, and lunges, which are very well capable of warming the muscles and enhancing flexibility.

- **Yoga and Pilates:** These are low-impact exercises that embody the objectives of flexibility, balance, and core strength as integral to maintaining mobility. It has also been indicated that yoga can have a positive effect on reducing stress and improving joint health. Peptide therapy will enable faster recovery from these workouts and hence give good long-term results.

- **Foam Rolling and Stretching:** Regular foam rolling and static stretches after exercise will help release tension from the muscles and avoid tightness. Both are important in maintaining mobility. Peptides such as BPC-157 speed up the healing process for soft tissues, making these techniques of recovery even more effective.

II. Functional Strength: Exercises to Maintain Independence

Functional strength exercises involve motions that can be applied to real-life activities and are necessary to maintain independence throughout the years. Peptides lessen recovery time and inflammation so that you can be more active and strong in your later years.

- **Bodyweight Exercises:** Exercises like squats, push-ups, and lunges are supposed to strengthen the muscles one engages in daily. Peptides will help your muscle repair and recovery from such workouts, enabling you to do them as frequently as possible without weariness or injury.

- **Core Training:** Core training will provide stability and balance to your body and even develop overall stength.

The plank, Russian twists, and leg raises will build up core strength to prevent back pain and improve your posture.

How to Create a Sustainable Fitness Routine Post- 60 Days

As you approach the end of your 60-day peptide therapy blueprint, it becomes increasingly important that you implement a long-term, sustainable pattern of fitness that will support the gains you have achieved through peptide therapy. Though peptides are indeed capable of helping with speedier recoveries and muscle gain right at the start, building upon these requires persistence and balance in your fitness routine.

I. Balanced Workout Schedule: Strength, Cardio, and Mobility Combined

Your training program should be a further balance of strength, cardiovascular exercise, and mobility work. In this respect, one should aim for a weekly schedule that covers:

- **3- 4** strength training sessions focused on the major large muscle groups such as the thighs, calf, abdominal muscles, back muscles, trapezius, triceps, and biceps.

- **2- 3** cardio sessions that combine HIIT and steady-state exercise.

- **1- 2** mobility sessions dedicated to flexibility, yoga, or dynamic stretching.

A balance between them will help you retain the strength, endurance, and flexibility that you have gained in the first 60 days and turn it into a long-term process.

II. Cycling Peptides for Continued Results

While one can cycle peptides after 60 days, it is very important to note that results are maintained through regular, balanced exercise, proper nutrition, and adequate sleep. Depending on one's fitness and health goals, one can continue using peptides to enhance recovery, improve cognitive functions, and anti-aging. However, cycling the peptides in 3 to 6-month intervals may avoid desensitization and let you maintain the benefits in the long run.

III. Preventing Overtraining and Burnout

One of the keys to a sustainable fitness routine is in avoiding overtraining and subsequent burnout. While peptides hasten recovery and diminish fatigue, one still needs to listen to their body and allow time for rest. Overtraining may lead to injuries, less motivation, and generally poor long-term results.

- **Rest Days:** Incorporate at least 1-2 rest days during the week to let the muscles recover and also avoid mental burnout.

- **Monitor Your Progress:** Chart your workouts and recovery times, along with your general physical feelings. If you encounter lingering fatigue, soreness, or lack of motivation, try dialing down your workout intensity or adding additional rest days.

A well-rounded exercise program individually designed for peptide therapy will maximize your capacity and return on muscular strength, cardiovascular health, mobility, and longevity. While the initial 60-day blueprint was instructive, it is important to create a long-term vision for a fitness program that would further solidify the gains created through peptide therapy. To that end, adding strengthening, cardiovascular exercises, and mobility work into a comprehensive, long-term regimen will promote vitality, physical fitness, and independence with aging.

Part 5:

Long-Term Health and Future Applications

Chapter 14

Maintaining Your Results for Life

As you reach the final stages of your 60-day journey into peptide therapy, attention shifts to how well you will sustain these transformative results. Peptide therapy has its great benefits, but it's exactly how you'll integrate these improvements into daily life that will ensure the long-term success of the therapy. The purpose of this chapter is to identify how one can keep the results for life through continuing peptide therapy responsibly, engaging in ongoing fitness, and lifestyle changes; and taking a long-term peptide protocol to maintain health.

Long-Term Peptide Protocols for Health Maintenance

As you transcend the 60-day peptide therapy program, one of the important ways to support your health improvements will be through taking on long-term peptide protocols. The peptides you've used thus far, BPC-157 for tissue repair and CJC-1295 for growth hormone release, have assisted your body in recovery, regeneration, and rejuvenation. However, in the long run, these will need to be used in cycles. Cyclical use of peptides avoids the development of tolerance to their actions in your body. This means using peptides for some time, usually 3-6 months, before you go on break for 1-2 months to allow the system to reset. In this way, they remain potent and do not develop side effects associated with their continuous administration.

The stacking of peptides is another method wherein multiple areas of health are targeted simultaneously. For instance, GHK-Cu is combined for skin rejuvenation with IGF-1, which helps in muscle recovery and growth; thus, overall health improvement is achieved. Generally speaking, peptide stacking should be done upon consultation with a healthcare professional for safety and effectiveness. It is important to continue monitoring through regular health assessments - including blood tests for hormone levels and liver function - for the assurance of beneficial and safe long-term use. With the institution of these protocols and follow-up close monitoring, you will be able to sustain the vitality, cognitive function, and physical recovery attributed to peptide therapy.

How to Continue Peptide Therapy Responsibly After 60 Days

Peptide therapy, if done responsibly, is both effective and safe even beyond the initial 60 days of continuation. The key to this lies in making sure you source your peptides from reputable suppliers since the market is sometimes not regulated. There are several online sources that are not verified selling counterfeit or low-quality peptide products. The best way to go about this is by working with licensed healthcare providers or pharmacies that specialize in peptide therapies for pure and high-quality peptides. These are also the providers to help tune your dosage and choose the most appropriate peptides based on ongoing needs.

It is important to talk to your healthcare professional regularly so you can adjust the therapy accordingly. Your body's needs will change over time, and so too should your peptide regimen. Follow-ups allow personalized guidance on peptide dosing, cycling, and combinations. This is very important, especially when you add new peptides to your regimen or change your goals. Measuring health metrics such as muscle mass, cognitive performance, and skin quality will give you an overview of how well one's body is responding to the peptides. With responsible peptide therapy for an extended period and under professional medical advice, you are going to have all the benefits while trying to reduce the risks associated with the therapy.

Integrating Peptide Therapy with Ongoing Fitness and Lifestyle Changes

Peptide therapy is most effective in the setting of a holistic lifestyle that includes regular exercise, proper nutrition, stress management, and adequate sleep. During peptide therapy, you should maintain an exercise program that helps promote what the peptides do for you. Resistance training should be at the heart of your workout program since it encourages the growth and recovery of muscles. Resistance training 3-4 days a week will help you maintain your muscle mass, strength, and resilience. Cardio exercises will also be necessary, either in the form of steady-state running or HIIT, for support of cardiovascular health, burning fat, and enhancing the complementary peptide effects to build muscle.

The other important factor is your diet that will help to maintain and enhance the results of peptide therapy. Continue with the high-protein intake; make sure your body is full of amino acids needed to build and repair muscle tissues. Adding these anti-inflammatory foods, like leafy vegetables, berries, and omega-3 fatty fish, may reduce inflammation, and it can also help in overall health. Additional supplementation of collagen and antioxidants, which would help skin elasticity and prevent oxidative stress, respectively, may enhance the benefits already seen by peptides such as GHK-Cu.

Finally, managing your stress and optimizing your sleep is fundamental to long-term success with peptide therapy. Chronic stress raises cortisol levels which can negate the benefits of peptides - especially those working for muscle growth and fat loss. Practice mindfulness, meditation, or yoga daily to help manage your stress levels and facilitate your body's recovery processes. Equally important is getting 7-9 hours of quality sleep each night, with peptides such as CJC-1295 and BPC-157 being most effective in deep sleep when the body naturally repairs itself. Thus, incorporating peptide therapy into an overall lifestyle approach that also includes regular exercise, proper nutrition, stress management, and quality sleep will allow you to sustain the benefits of peptides and further optimize overall health and vitality.

Chapter 15

Innovations in Peptide Therapy

The Future of Peptide Research and New Developments
Peptide therapy is a constantly developing field in medicine; therefore, it has a promising future in the optimization of human health. The current research into peptides aims at the discovery of new peptides and improving their modes of administration to have more specific and effective treatments. Advances in biotechnology and genetic research place peptide therapy at the front line in the field of personalized medicine. Now, researchers can have far better insights into the exact mechanisms by which certain peptides act through cellular pathways, and thus possibilities are opening for the creation of custom-tailored peptide treatments, based on an individual's genetics, his lifestyle, and particular health needs.

The other major developments in prospect involve the synthesis of peptides with even longer half-lives and with greater specificity, targeting a particular cell or tissue. That means that peptides can be designed to provide longer-lasting effects with fewer injections. This is going to reduce the need for frequent dosing and will make peptide therapy more convenient for patients. In addition, current research into the application of peptide nanotechnology has indicated that the combination of peptides with nanoparticles can remarkably improve their delivery in the body. This, in turn, can provide better absorption and effectiveness of peptides in order for them to reach some targets more effectively.

With these newer developments, peptide therapy soon may be a big part of preventive medicine itself and thus forestall the development of, or completely avoid, age-related diseases. Clinical trials are underway with peptides in conditions as diverse as Alzheimer's, cancer, and cardiovascular diseases. Further research in these directions will doubtless bring about a future wherein peptides not only serve in symptomatic treatment but powerfully act in the prevention of diseases and attainment of longevity.

Emerging Peptides for Longevity, Disease Prevention, and Cognitive Enhancement

Emerging peptides are showing promise beyond what current peptide therapy covers in the areas of enhancing longevity, preventing chronic diseases, and improving cognitive function. One of the most exciting peptides coming into prominence is MOTS-c, a mitochondrial-derived peptide that has shown great potential in healthy aging through improvement in metabolic function and protection against age-related diseases. It activates pathways that are associated with improvements in insulin sensitivity, fat metabolism, and the production of energy. Thus, MOTS-c has great potential for the treatment of metabolic disorders related to diabetes and obesity apart from its overall enhancement of vitality.

Another very promising peptide is KPV, an anti-inflammatory peptide, which helps with the lessening of chronic inflammation at the cellular level.

Chronic inflammation is associated with most age-related diseases, including arthritis, cardiovascular disease, and neurodegenerative conditions such as Alzheimer's. Targeting inflammation, KPV opens up avenues not only for managing the symptoms but possibly even delaying the onset of such diseases.

Another fast-growing area of application for peptides is cognitive enhancement. Currently, some peptides like Dihexa and RG3 are being investigated for neuroprotective purposes; early studies have shown the improvement of memory formation, cognitive function, and synaptic plasticity. These peptides have now shown promise in treating neurodegenerative diseases like Alzheimer's and Parkinson's and even enhancing cognition in healthy individuals. In the future, we are going to see even more peptides targeted at keeping the brain healthy as people age.

How to Stay Informed About the Latest Peptide Innovations

Because of the extremely rapid pace of unfolding research on peptides, anyone interested in optimizing their health through peptide therapy would be well-served by knowing recent happenings. Also, one of the best ways to keep updated is by reading peer-reviewed and reputable current medical journals and clinical research publications. Journals such as Nature Reviews Drug Discovery, The Journal of Peptide Science, and Frontiers in Aging Neuroscience are among the most frequent publishers in peer-reviewed studies related to the latest peptide research.

These publications often include insight into ongoing clinical trials, breakthrough discoveries, and new uses of peptides in medicine.

Another prized source of knowledge is attendance at anti-aging and regenerative medicine medical conferences on peptide therapy. The World Congress on Anti-Aging Medicine and the Peptide Summit are the pinnacles where leading researchers, clinicians, and experts meet and discuss discoveries and practical applications of peptides. Events like this allow the opportunity to network with industry leaders and understand future peptide protocols directly from the source.

Besides, close cooperation with a professional healthcare provider specialized in peptide therapy will give you access to the most updated knowledge. Many peptide specialists take part in clinical research or maintain close connections with such works. You will not only be constantly improving your peptide regimen through regular consultations with them but also get acquainted with new peptides coming up that may be useful for your long-term health objectives.

Finally, following reputable online forums and social platforms that deal with peptide therapy proves to be invaluable on an informatory level. Websites like Peptide Sciences and The International Peptide Society have regular updates of new peptide products available, research findings, and educational resources for practitioners and patients alike. In this regard, when one is updated with these resources, they are in a better position to adapt and integrate into their regimen state-of-the-art peptides as they become available, hence ensuring they continue benefiting from the latest developments in this fast-evolving field.

Conclusion

Chapter 16

Your 60-Day Transformation: What's Next?

Celebrating Your Success: Reflecting on Your Health Journey

Coming towards the end of your 60-day peptide therapy now would be a good time to give a rundown on how well you have been doing. These last couple of months have been a journey of self-discovery through regulated improvements in your vitality, longevity, cognitive function, and physical recovery. The changes, whether subtle or overwhelming, attest to the commitment you've shown toward securing better health and unlocking every potentiality within peptide therapy.

Take a minute to enjoy your success. Refer back to the particular goals you wished to achieve at the start of this journey. Have you noticed improvements in skin elasticity and skin glow? Your muscles, after working out, recover faster and feel stronger. Your mind is sharper; it's more capable of dealing with challenges with much greater focus and ease. These are tangible results that serve as milestones of your progress and show just how effective peptides can be when used strategically. Success, in this respect, encompasses much more than the physical changes a person can observe but also the positive ways in which the mindset changes. In the course of this journey, you have identified the ways of caring for your well-being, from fine-tuning nutrition to adopting exercise routines that best complement your peptide protocol.

These are gains that reach beyond the 60-day mark, building blocks for a more energetic and healthy life.

Perhaps most relevant is recognition of the personal growth you have undergone. With each modification in lifestyle, every new approach you learned and adopted to handle life's stressors, with the fine-tuning of food in your diet, you became stronger in your resolve to take responsibility for your health. You have invested knowledge and experience in peptide therapy and have committed yourself to consistency with your regimen; this will pay off for many years to come. This success that you're celebrating isn't just about what you've done over the last two months; it's about what you've learned about your body, your health, and your capacity for change.

Planning for Future Peptide Use and Continued Health Improvements

As you move beyond this initial phase of peptide therapy, you start to wonder how to maintain those results and plan for continued improvements. The good news with peptide therapy is that it is not a one-time intervention but rather an evolving strategy that can be tailored to your ever-changing health needs. Now that you have seen and harnessed the power of peptides firsthand, you can begin to contemplate how to use them in a long-term strategy in respect to overall health. First, you need to consider what peptides seemed to be working best. Through this 60-day process, you tried a series of peptides that were targeted to help with anti-aging, recovery muscles, cognitive enhancement, and general wellness.

Identify which peptides yield better results and continue with these as part of a maintenance program. For example, if BPC-157 and GHK-Cu were highly effective in giving good skin health and low inflammation, one might consider continuing administration at a much lower dose to maintain the positive effects of the peptides. Similarly, peptides such as IGF-1 and CJC-1295, which are targeted at muscle recovery and strength gains, can be cycled on and off based on your workout routine.

It is equally OK to continue working with a healthcare professional who has experience in peptide therapy. This will ensure that your use of peptides remains safe and effective, even if your health needs change over time. Regular blood work, hormone panels, and health check-ups can guide an adjustment in your protocol to make sure the peptides are working harmoniously with your body's biochemistry. This also means you get to have the latest state of progress in peptides and studies introduced to you by your health expert, which might complement what you are taking.

In addition to peptides, continuing all lifestyle changes you have made regarding nutrition, exercise, sleep, and stress will continue to enhance your results. Consider setting new health objectives for your future: improving your cardiovascular health, enhancing cognitive function even more, or promoting longevity. As you move further in this direction, remember that the peptides are only one tool in your utility belt; it's their integration with the holistic approach to health that will make the greatest benefits long-term.

Final Thoughts on Achieving a Longer, Healthier, and More Vital Life

The 60-day peptide therapy journey is just the beginning of what can be a lifelong commitment toward the optimization of health, vitality, and longevity. Peptide therapy can be a very advanced, scientifically supported means to improve many aspects of your physical and mental well-being. However, the real magic happens when peptides are used in concert with other healthy strategies. Blending good nutrition, regular exercise, sound sleep, and controlled stress with peptide use will set one up for success and long-term vitality.

One critical takeaway from this journey is that longevity is not just about living longer; it's about living better. Living longer and healthier requires a continuing commitment to informed decision-making, and peptide therapy is one of the most promising tools available to support that commitment. Be it for youthful skin, muscle recovery, improved cognitive function, or any number of other uses currently being researched to help your body fight off age-related degeneration, the possible benefits are profound.

It is, however, important to note that peptides will only work properly when their consumption is considerably regular and well strategically managed. Peptide therapy is not a quick fix but rather a continued supportive process of your body's natural functions and cellular health. As time progresses and with ongoing research, other peptides and protocols will unfold, thus opening more doors to the opportunities available toward enhancing one's health and extending vitality.

Moving forward, just remember that optimal health is in constant flux and evolution. Stay open to changes as new information becomes available, and stay ahead of the curve with your health. Make sure you have all the support you need, whether it be with the right medical professionals, personal trainers, nutritionists, or wellness communities, to make educated decisions that align with your goals.

Your 60-day peptide therapy transformation is just the beginning of living your life to the fullest, as the most vibrant version of you. You now have all the tools, knowledge, and experience in store to keep bettering your health for many years to come. Keep learning, remain disciplined, but above all else, stay focused on what's most important: the prize of a life teeming with energy, vitality, and good health. Peptide therapy has unlocked the door to living longer and healthier, and with the right strategies in place, the best is yet to come.

Appendices

Meal Plan and Exercise Templates

Nutrition and exercise go hand in hand to optimize the benefits of your peptide therapy. Here are some sample meal plans and an exercise template you can easily follow for longevity, muscle recovery, cognition, and general health.

Sample Meal Plan for Peptide Optimization:

Breakfast:

- Protein smoothie with whey or plant-based protein, spinach, berries, and flaxseeds.

- 1 boiled egg or a small serving of nuts for additional protein and healthy fats.

- Herbal tea or decaf coffee with a minimum amount of sugar.

Lunch:

- Grilled salmon or chicken breast, served with quinoa and steamed broccoli.

- Mixed green salad with olive oil and apple cider vinegar, topped with seeds for added nutrition.

- Water to drink, with slices of lemon or cucumber in the water.

Snack:

- A handful of almonds or walnuts.

- 1 cup sliced vegetables (carrots/cucumber) with hummus to dip into

Dinner:

- Grass-fed beef or tofu stir-fry with bell peppers, onions, and mushrooms.

- Serve with sweet potatoes or brown rice.

- Water or herbal tea for hydration and digestive ease.

Before Bed:

- Chamomile tea for extra restful sleep and relaxation.

- Greek yogurt or cottage cheese with a drizzle of honey for protein and digestive health.

Sample Exercise Plan for Peptide-Enhanced Recovery and Longevity:

Strength Training (3x per week):

- **Day 1 (Upper Body):** push-ups, dumbbell bench press, bicep curls, shoulder press, pull-ups.

- **Day 2, (Lower Body):** squats, deadlifts, lunges, calf raises, glute bridges.

- **Day 3, (Full Body):** deadlifts, kettlebell swings, burpees, renegade rows, planks.

Cardio, 2x a week:

- **Day 1:** 20-30 minutes of steady-state cardio: cycling, jogging, or swimming.

- **Day 2:** HIIT, High-Intensity Interval Training- alternating between 30 seconds of sprinting with 90 seconds of walking for 15-20 minutes.

Flexibility and Recovery, 2x a week:

- Yoga or Pilates sessions focused on stretching major muscle groups.

- After every workout, 15-20 minutes for recovery through foam rolling or deep stretching.

Glossary of Key Terms in Peptide Science

Peptides: Small chains of amino acids that are linked through peptide bonds. Peptides act as signaling molecules within the body, influencing many biological activities, including tissue repair, hormone production, and immune function.

BPC-157: This is by far one of the most powerful peptides with the most impressive healing capabilities, especially for muscle and tissue-related issues. This peptide has potential applications in accelerating the recovery process and enhancing gut health status.

GHK-Cu: It is a copper-binding peptide that facilitates regeneration and anti-aging. It stimulates collagen production and helps in wound healing and skin health.

CJC-1295: Growth hormone-releasing hormone analog (GHRH) which improves levels of growth hormone, therefore promoting fat loss, muscle gain, and cellular repair.

IGF-1 (Insulin-like Growth Factor 1): The peptide mimics the action of insulin and bears a very important role in growth and development. IGF-1 improves myogenesis, recovery, and cellular regeneration.

Cerebrolysin: A peptide nootropic drug with neuroprotective and cognitive-enhancing action, which promotes brain health, enhances memory, and may help in the prevention of neurodegenerative disorders.

Dihexa: This is a peptide designed for the enhancement of cognitive function, neural repair, and restoration of neuronal tissue. It is also well recognized for enhancing learning and memory capabilities and the health of the brain generally.

Peptide Cycling: The administration of peptides for a period of time, followed by a period of rest, to avoid desensitization and maintain effectiveness.

GHS- Growth Hormone Secretagogues; peptides that stimulate the secretion of growth hormone in the pituitary gland and are responsible for anything from muscle growth and fat loss to recovery in general.

Third-Party Testing: A process in which peptides are tested for their quality and purity by an independent laboratory so that standards regarding safety and effectiveness can be met.

Bioavailability: Refers to the extent a peptide or a medication is absorbed into the bloodstream and is, therefore, available to be utilized by the body. Many peptides depend on certain routes of administration to maintain optimum bioavailability.